Hands On

Developing your differential diagnostic skills

A workbook for demonstrating
continuing professional development

Simon Browning DO Cert Ed

tfm publishing Ltd, Castle Hill Barns, Harley, Nr Shrewsbury, SY5 6LX, UK
Tel: +44 (0)1952 510061; Fax: +44 (0)1952 510192
E-mail: nikki@tfmpublishing.com; Web site: www.tfmpublishing.com

Design and layout: Nikki Bramhill
Illustrations: Simon Browning

Copyright © 2006 tfm publishing Ltd

ISBN 1 903378 43 5

NOTICE

Printed by Gutenberg Press Ltd., Gudja Road, Tarxien, PLA 19, Malta

Tel: +356 21897037; Fax: +356 21800069

Contents

Introduction

This book is ideally suited for a therapist's continuing professional development portfolio, whether they are a practising osteopath, chiropractor, physiotherapist or professional physical therapist. Continuing professional development is designed to encourage the practitioner to demonstrate an enquiring mind, refresh their knowledge base and reflect upon their clinical practice. This workbook, by focusing upon the process of reaching a diagnosis, will enable the practitioner to demonstrate all three aspects of CPD, either by working alone or with others. It follows the complete consultation process of not only a new patient but also the old patient who, it should be remembered, can develop medical problems between consultations. Many patients will be of an age when the early signs or symptoms of systemic disease first become apparent, often being put down to 'getting older' or their 'time of life'. As many of these patients will not have seen their doctor for many years, it is your professional responsibility to be alert to the early signs and symptoms of the common systemic diseases, to know how to complete a simple screening examination, and to assess the potential seriousness of the underlying condition to ensure the patient receives the appropriate treatment or advice.

The workbook is divided into sections, each dealing with a different aspect of the consultation process covering the general observation of the patient, aspects of the case history, physical evaluation and specific systemic system examination procedures. To ensure the full differential diagnostic process is covered and recorded, it is necessary occasionally to ask very simplistic or basic questions. By answering these an experienced practitioner will challenge and reflect upon their personal diagnostic criteria, while the less experienced will reinforce their knowledge gained during training. In addition there is some repetition of the common signs and symptoms of systemic disease; however, this has been kept to a minimum. For ease and simplicity, the broad age groupings: 0-20, 20-40, 40-60 and 60+, have been adopted when considering the onset for a particular condition, sign or symptom. The final section contains sample answers which are intentionally brief and should be used as a starting point for further thought, reading or research after writing your first complete answer in the workbook.

You may wish to work steadily through the workbook completing a section at a time or focus upon specific areas that you have identified as requiring revision. Once completed, it may be prudent to return to the workbook after 8-12 months and review your answers based upon your most recent experiences from clinical practice, reflecting on how your new knowledge base has modified your clinical practice. Throughout the book are CPD record sheets. These will enable you to record the time devoted to each section, either working by oneself or with others. The space at the foot of the page can be used to identify areas that require further study, when this was completed, and the time taken.

To help you with your research before answering the questions in the workbook, I would recommend in particular the following internet sites:

General information   http://medicine.ucsd.edu/clinicalmed/introduction.htm

Rheumatology   http://www.ucl.ac.uk/~regfjxe/Studentinfo2.htm

Cardiovascular   http://www.blaufuss.org
http://www.med.ucla.edu/wilkes/inex.htm

Respiratory   http://www.umshp.org/rt/sounds/sounds.html
http://medocs.ucdavis.edu/IMD/420C/sounds/lngsound.htm

In addition, my first book, *Hands On: A Clinical Companion. Steps to confidence in musculoskeletal diagnosis* (ISBN 1 903378 30 3; tfm publishing), will be helpful in the musculoskeletal section. For the other sections, I would recommend any medical textbook or clinical methods book. I have found the following to be clear and easy to read:

1) *An introduction to the symptoms and signs of clinical medicine*, Arnold (ISBN 0340732075)

2) *Davidson's Principles and Practice of Medicine*, Churchill Livingstone (ISBN 0443059446)

3) *Aids to the examination of the peripheral nervous system*, Churchill Livingstone (ISBN 0702025127)

4) *Further neurological examination made easy*, Churchill Livingstone (ISBN 0443074208)

Simon Browning
January 2006

Acknowledgements

I would like to thank the College of Osteopaths Educational Trust for allowing me to use and develop the ideas, themes and format from coursework I wrote for their undergraduate programme in the production of this workbook. In addition I would like to thank Robin Kirk, Bob Burge and Fiona Hamilton for their help, advice and comments. Finally, I am indebted to Carol West, a qualified osteopath with experience in publishing, who proof-read the entire workbook with a very critical eye.

Section 1

General observation of the patient

Although we may be reluctant to admit it, we all make assumptions of the next patient waiting in reception. These may be based purely on appearance and age, previous encounters and their response to treatment, or some 'sixth sense' or 'gut instinct'. In this section the emphasis is upon what the practitioner, if alert, can observe and what those subtle and occasionally not-so-subtle signs can add to the consultation process. They may suggest a musculoskeletal problem, an underlying clinical or sub-clinical disease process or absolutely nothing at all.

Whilst observing the patient in the waiting room, it is occasionally possible to make an assessment of not only their physical health (musculoskeletal and systemic systems) but also their psychosocial health.

1.1 Musculoskeletal system

By noting the obvious: the patient's apparent age, sex, posture, and mobility, an initial guess of the type of musculoskeletal problem they may have can be made.

In the following box list what general musculoskeletal conditions could be present when considering these obvious features. Are there any other observations that you would find helpful?

> Patient's age
>
> Patient's gender
>
> Patient's posture
>
> Accompanying support aids
>
> Others

It is important to remember that the overt signs may be from old problems and that the patient could actually be consulting you regarding something totally different.

1.2 Systemic system

The signs of underlying systemic disease can be overt or subtle. In the following boxes predictors of disease and signs of disease are noted. Indicate which system or systems are affected.

Specific predictors	Which system(s) affected
Patient smokes	
Other predictors	

Specific signs	Which system(s) affected
Facial skin colour:	
yellowish hue	
red/ruddy	
blue tinge to lips	
Unsuitable clothing considering the ambient outside temperature	
Constant blowing of nose	
Other signs	

1.3 Psychosocial issues

The demeanour of the patient may give an insight to the degree of strain that they are under, and whether it has affected them in the short or long term. In the following box indicate what signs of psychological strain can be apparent. State if it is possible to determine if the signs are due to short- or long-term psychosocial issues.

1.4 Other signs or predictors

Whilst escorting the patient to the treatment room, assisting them with their coat and watching them sit down, other signs or predictors of underlying musculoskeletal or systemic disease can be discretely observed.

In the following box (continued on the next page) indicate what systemic and musculoskeletal conditions are suggested by the six specific observations listed; for example, breathlessness may suggest a rib problem or asthma. In addition, add other observations, noting which system could be affected.

Signs	Musculoskeletal system	Systemic systems
Breathlessness		
Difficulty in sitting		

Signs	Musculoskeletal system	Systemic systems
Altered gait		
Poor mobility of specific joint(s)		
Poor mobility in general		
Unsteadiness		
Other signs		

Continuing Professional Development
Record Sheet

To assist when submitting your CPD summary or for your portfolio, please use this page to identify the time spent working through this section.

Hands On: developing your differential diagnostic skills.

Name: ………….. CPD year: ……...............……

Date	Pages covered	Number of CPD hours		Venue / people involved
		Learning by oneself	Learning with others	

Date	Area	Identified areas for further study		Venue / people involved
		Learning by oneself	Learning with others	

Signature: ……………………......………… Date: ………..............

Aspects of the case history process

The aim of undertaking the case history process is to enable the practitioner to reach an initial hypothesis that identifies the cause of the patient's symptoms. To reach this goal six different aspects of the patient should be considered before the physical examination is undertaken. These aspects will concern the symptoms from musculoskeletal or systemic conditions and their physiological effects. The six aspects are:

1) General musculoskeletal signs and symptoms.
2) Predisposing and precipitating factors, physical and physiological.
3) Symptoms referred from the systemic system.
4) Specific joint and joint complex signs and symptoms.
5) General health indicators and issues.
6) Past medical history indicators and issues.

2.1 General musculoskeletal signs and symptoms

Most patients presenting at your practice will complain of an unpleasant sensation, generally an ache or a pain. Indicate in the following box how you would define the following descriptors for pain.

Acute pain

Sub-acute pain

Chronic pain

The pain sensation can be modified from within the neurological system or by internal or external factors. In the following box indicate how you believe this modification occurs, giving examples where the sensation is reduced or enhanced: within the neurological pathways, within the body (internal factors) or from local environmental factors (external factors).

Neurological pathways

Internal factors

External factors

Many patients suffer with chronic or recurrent conditions. What specific factors, physical and psychological, can modify the pain felt at the initial episode of the condition to that felt after many recurrences of the problem?

Much has been written about psychological factors and their effect on, in particular, the rate of recovery from either an acute or a long-term musculoskeletal problem. The following books are recommended:

1) Waddell G. *The Back Pain Revolution*. London: Churchill Livingstone, 1998 (ISBN 0443 060398).
2) Main CC, Spanswick CJ. *Pain Management*. London: Churchill Livingstone, 1999 (ISBN 0443 056838).

To ensure that specific conditions are not overlooked during the musculoskeletal differential diagnostic process, the prudent practitioner would question if any of the symptoms are associated with an undiagnosed physical or systemic problem. The following simple checklist may assist in identifying potential physical or systemic problems related to the patient's age at the time of original onset of the symptoms. Does the patient have:

- a congenital or developmental condition?
- a rheumatological condition (specific, vague or poorly understood)?
- an underlying primary or secondary neoplastic condition?
- a referral from a specific system?
- a condition related to the degree of degenerative changes present (musculoskeletal, systemic or neurological)?
- a musculoskeletal condition?

In the following box list any general signs or symptoms from the case history that would suggest the patient has one of the following conditions.

Congenital	
Developmental	
Rheumatological	
Underlying neoplastic	
Referral from a specific system	
Degenerative	
Musculoskeletal	

2.1 General musculoskeletal signs

2.1.1 Local musculoskeletal tissue

Identifying the local primary tissue(s) causing symptoms will assist in generating an initial hypothesis. Five specific tissues for spinal pain are often considered: ligament, muscle, bone, facet and disc. For the peripheral joints, the five specific tissues would be ligament, muscle, bone, joint and fat pad / bursa.

In the following box indicate what you consider to be the primary aggravating and relieving features for each of the identified tissues. Add any other tissues you consider relevant.

Tissue causing symptoms	Aggravating movements / activities	Relieving movements / activities
Muscle		
Ligament		
Facet / joint		
Disc		
Bursa		
Fat pad		
Bone		
Other tissues		

In every presentation the patient's tissue state will be altered and in most cases some degree of inflammatory response will be present. How will this inflammatory response modify the presenting symptoms?

Tissue / state	Modify symptoms by
Acute inflammation (<6 weeks)	
Sub-acute inflammation	
Chronic inflammation (>6 weeks)	

2.1.2 Rheumatological and systemic conditions

The term 'rheumatological condition' is used here in its broadest sense to encompass the classical medical rheumatological / autoimmune conditions (sero-positive and sero-negative) and also vague and poorly understood conditions or syndromes such as fibromyalgia and myalgic encephalomyelitis (ME).

Medical rheumatological / autoimmune conditions

In the following box list any indicators, signs or symptoms present in the case history that would suggest that the patient had an underlying rheumatological condition. At this stage it is important to identify only the general signs and symptoms, not the specifics of any one condition.

Indicators
General symptoms
General signs

Whilst taking the patient's case history, the pattern of the joint pain or associated systemic symptoms can alert you to the possible presence of a rheumatological condition. In the following box indicate what conditions are suggested by the patterns of pain listed.

Joint pain	Named rheumatological conditions	Joints affected	Systemic symptoms / signs
Monoarthritic pain			
Symmetrical polyarthritic pain			
Asymmetrical polyarthritic pain			

2.1.2 Rheumatological and systemic conditions

Vague and poorly understood conditions

Medicine is not a precise science and there are many aspects or facets of a patient's health or state of disease that are poorly understood. One easy way of labelling any vague and variable combination of musculoskeletal and systemic symptoms is by utilising the terms fibromyalgia and ME. Before any patient can be given such a label, all possible pathological causes for the symptoms must first be ruled out. In the following box list your personal diagnostic criteria for the identified conditions, together with an indication of the medical conditions that would need to be ruled out. Add any other similar conditions.

'Syndrome'	Identifying symptoms or signs	Differential diagnosis
ME		
Fibromyalgia		
Irritable bowel syndrome (IBS)		
Others		

Systemic conditions

There are many systemic conditions that can affect the joints and have associated systemic symptoms / signs.

In the following two boxes list the conditions you know naming each affected joint, together with the associated systemic symptoms / signs.

Joint pain	Named systemic conditions	Joints affected	Systemic symptoms / signs
Monoarthritic pain			

Joint pain	Named systemic conditions	Joints affected	Systemic symptoms / signs
Symmetrical polyarthritic pain			
Asymmetrical polyarthritic pain			

2.2 Predisposing and precipitating factors, physical and physiological

During the consultation it is helpful to review the various predisposing and precipitating factors for the patient's problems that have become apparent by this stage of the patient / practitioner encounter. These can be physical (short or long term) or physiological (short or long term).

2.2.1 Physical factors

There are many outside factors that can affect our patients; however, it is how the individual patient reacts to those variable factors that will determine not only rate of recovery but also duration and severity of symptoms.

In the following two boxes list some short- and long-term physical factors.

Short-term factors

Long-term factors

Many patients with chronic medical or genetic problems will present with musculoskeletal symptoms. In the following box several conditions are suggested which require special precautions or care to be taken. Indicate what these precautions are and why they are necessary.

Condition	Precautions taken and why
Rheumatoid arthritis	
Marfan's syndrome	
Down's syndrome	
Turner's syndrome	
Graves' disease	
Other conditions	

When long-term physical, psychological or medical problems exist, the patient will probably be on long-term medication. In the following box indicate how different common types of long-term medication will affect the body's physiological response to injury. Steroid therapy is suggested; add any other medications that also modify this response.

Long-term oral steroid therapy

Other medication

2.2.2 *Physiological factors*

When the patient is faced with an emotionally stressful situation, what is the normal short-term physiological response to this 'stress' that occurs within their body?

Describe the effects of the response, from hypothalamus to end organ, listing the common signs or symptoms associated with this fight or flight reaction.

Previously, the body's physiological response to the fight or flight reaction was described. If the stressful situation does not resolve quickly, how will the body's internal response be modified? In the following box describe how the response is physiologically modified and how this will affect any physical signs and symptoms. Indicate the possible long-term effects on the body of this altered physiological response.

2.3 Symptoms referred from the systemic system

Many of the body's systems will tend to refer symptoms to specific areas of the skeleton. In the following box indicate where you expect each of the named systems to refer; there may be more than one referral site. If possible describe the nature of pain or symptoms, side commonly felt, common or classical aggravating and relieving factors.

System	Referral to	Nature of symptoms	Aggravated by	Relieved by
Cardiovascular				
Respiratory				
Upper digestive tract				
Small intestine				
Lower digestive tract				
Genitourinary				
Gynaecological				
Biliary				

Whilst taking the case history it is important, in addition to the above, to remember that named systemic disorders can give rise to musculoskeletal symptoms. In the box below list the systemic symptoms for the named conditions, indicating the joints commonly affected and the pattern of joint involvement (monoarthritic or polyarthritic, symmetrical or asymmetrical).

2.3 Symptoms

Condition	Systemic symptoms / signs	Joints affected	Joint pain pattern
Ulcerative colitis			
Crohn's disease			
IBS			
Other conditions			

In the following box list any other musculoskeletal or physical conditions (for example craniosacral imbalances) that can be associated with disorders in the systemic system. Indicate how the two, physical and visceral, are linked and how gross pathological causes of the symptoms are ruled out.

Neoplasms can occur at any age and may be the cause of the patient's presenting complaint. If a neoplasm is present, indicate the general signs / symptoms that may alert the practitioner.

In the following box indicate the age that the following common neoplastic changes occur: prostate, lung, breast, testicular, melanoma and large bowel. Add any other common cancers and the typical age of presentation.

Age	Named neoplasm	Typical presenting symptoms / signs
0-20		
20-40		
40-60		
60+		

Continuing Professional Development
Record Sheet

To assist when submitting your CPD summary or for your portfolio, please use this page to identify the time spent working through this section.

Hands On: developing your differential diagnostic skills.

Name: …………...……………………………………………………………...…………….. CPD year: ………...............……

Date	Pages covered	Number of CPD hours		Venue / people involved
		Learning by oneself	Learning with others	

Date	Area	Identified areas for further study		Venue / people involved
		Learning by oneself	Learning with others	

Signature: ………………………....…………… Date: ……………...........

2.4 Specific joint and joint complex signs and symptoms

On the following pages consider specific joints or joint complexes. Identify:

♦ musculoskeletal areas or systemic systems that can refer to the area;
♦ specific joint or systemic problems that occur local to the area;
♦ common musculoskeletal tissues that cause symptoms in the area.

2.4.1 Head and face

Head and face symptoms or headaches can originate from within the bony structures (the sinuses, middle or inner ear, the oral or nasal cavities, or cranial fascia), be associated with the local musculoskeletal system (temporomandibular joint [TMJ]), referred from another part of the musculoskeletal system, related to a rheumatological condition or referred from one of the body's other systems.

In the following box identify from where the pain or symptoms could be referred. One musculoskeletal area and two visceral areas that can refer to the head are suggested; list any other sites or conditions you can think of, together with a simple way of deciding from where the symptoms are being referred.

Referral site / condition	How to determine from where the symptoms could be referred
Musculoskeletal referral	
Cervical spine	
Rheumatological condition	
Visceral referral	
Cardiovascular system	
Digestive system	

What TMJ or other local musculoskeletal problem could give rise to head symptoms? In the following box list the conditions indicating the classical presenting symptom picture.

```



```

What ear problems could give rise to head symptoms? In the following box list named conditions for the outer, middle and inner ear, indicating the classical presenting symptom picture.

```



```

What facial and temporal problems could give rise to head symptoms? In the following box list any conditions (excluding the TMJ and cranial fascia) with their classical presenting symptom picture.

```



```

What cranial vault or cranial fascia problems could give rise to head symptoms? In the following box list any conditions with their classical presenting symptom picture.

```



```

2.4.1 Head and face

The patient's age, together with site, description or pattern of symptoms may suggest that a specific condition is present. Using the following boxes continue to list what you consider these possible conditions may be, together with the classical presenting symptoms.

Age of onset of head or face symptoms

0-20	
20-40	
40-60	
60+	

Site of head or face symptoms

Frontal	
Parietal	
Temporal	
Facial	
Occipital	

Description of head or face symptoms

Throbbing / pulsating	
Tight constricting band	
Constant dull ache / pain	

Pattern of head or face symptoms

Single episode	
Recurrent monthly	
Recurrent weekly	
Recurrent daily	
Night-time	
Early morning	
Afternoon / evening	
Specific event(s)	

2.4.2 Cervical spine and cervicothoracic junction

The terms cervical spine and cervicothoracic junction include the three different functional groups of vertebrae: the upper cervical complex, the cervical spine and the cervicothoracic junction.

When taking a case history, it is important to remember that the symptoms can be originating from any one of these three functional groups of vertebrae, associated with another part of the musculoskeletal system, related to a rheumatological condition or referred from one of the body's other systems.

In the following box identify from where the pain or symptoms could be referred. Two musculoskeletal areas and three visceral areas that can refer to the cervical spine are suggested; list any other sites or conditions you can think of, together with a simple way of deciding from where the symptoms are being referred.

Referral site / condition	How to determine from where the symptoms could be referred
Musculoskeletal referral Shoulder complex	
Upper ribs / thorax	
Rheumatological condition	

Visceral referral
  Cardiovascular system
  (shoulder, neck,
  upper thorax)	

Biliary system (right shoulder)	
Digestive system (retrosternal)	

The patient's age when the symptoms originally began may suggest specific underlying conditions. Using the following age groupings and headings, list what you consider these possible conditions may be.

0-20	Congenital	
	Developmental	
	Rheumatological	

20-40	Congenital	
	Developmental	
	Postural / occupational	
	Rheumatological	

40-60	Hormonal / age	
	Postural / occupational	
	Rheumatological	

60+	Degenerative	
	Hormonal / age	
	Rheumatological	

Generally, musculoskeletal symptoms occur following a specific event or gradually for no apparent reason over a period of days, months or years.

If the onset was sudden, resulting from one notable incident, suggest causes for the patient's symptoms bearing in mind your experience.

For the above indicate the primary tissues causing symptoms, together with your personal differential diagnostic rationale for selecting those tissues (aggravating and relieving features).

If the onset was for no apparent reason, suggest causes for the patient's symptoms bearing in mind your experience.

For the above indicate the primary tissues causing symptoms, together with your personal differential diagnostic rationale for selecting those tissues (aggravating and relieving features).

As the cervical spine is the final part of the spinal column, indicate what other musculoskeletal problems (either spinal or lower limb) could produce local cervical symptoms.

2.4.3 Thoracic cage

The term thoracic cage includes the thoracic vertebrae, ribs, costal cartilages and sternum.

When taking a case history, it is important to remember that the symptoms can be originating from the thoracic cage, associated with another part of the musculoskeletal system, related to a rheumatological condition or referred from the viscera, in particular the organs contained within the thoracic cage.

In the following box identify from where the pain or symptoms could be referred. Several visceral areas that can refer to the thoracic cage are suggested; list any other sites or conditions you can think of, together with a simple way of deciding from where the symptoms are being referred.

Referral site / condition	How to determine from where the symptoms could be referred
Musculoskeletal referral	
Rheumatological condition	
Visceral referral Cardiovascular system (left or right shoulder)	
Respiratory system (diaphragm [left or right shoulder])	
Biliary system (right shoulder)	
Renal system (left or right loin)	
Other (left shoulder) (generalised)	

2.4.3 Thoracic cage

In the thoracic cage, the site of symptoms as well as the descriptive terms used by the patient can assist in determining the organ involved.

In the following box several different organs have been suggested that can refer symptoms to the thoracic cage. Indicate the typical descriptive terms used by the patient to describe the pain experienced for each organ.

Organ	Descriptive terms used to describe the pain
Heart	
Digestive (oesophagus)	
Respiratory	
Biliary	

In addition the various organs / systems also refer to specific areas of the thoracic cage indicated below. Identify these in the following box.

Site of pain	Referring organ or system
Retrosternal	
Chest wall	
Upper thoracic cage	
Whole chest	

The patient's age when the symptoms originally began may suggest specific underlying conditions. Using the following age groupings and headings, list what you consider these possible conditions may be.

0-20	Congenital	
	Developmental	
	Rheumatological	

20-40	Congenital	
	Developmental	
	Postural / occupational	
	Rheumatological	

40-60	Hormonal / age	
	Postural / occupational	
	Rheumatological	

60+	Degenerative	
	Hormonal / age	
	Rheumatological	

2.4.3 Thoracic cage

Generally, musculoskeletal symptoms occur following a specific event or gradually for no apparent reason over a period of days, months or years.

If the onset was sudden, resulting from one notable incident, suggest causes for the patient's symptoms bearing in mind your experience.

For the above indicate the primary tissues causing symptoms, together with your personal differential diagnostic rationale for selecting those tissues (aggravating and relieving features).

If the onset was for no apparent reason, suggest causes for the patient's symptoms bearing in mind your experience.

For the above indicate the primary tissues causing symptoms, together with your personal differential diagnostic rationale for selecting those tissues (aggravating and relieving features).

Indicate what spinal changes or named pathological conditions could occur in the thoracic spine of a postmenopausal woman or elderly male patient.

2.4.4 Lumbar spine

The lumbar spine refers to the spinal area between and including the lumbosacral and thoracolumbar junctions.

When taking a case history, it is important to remember that the symptoms can be originating from the lumbar spine, associated with another part of the musculoskeletal system, related to a rheumatological condition or referred from one of the body's other systems.

In the following box identify from where the pain or symptoms could be referred. Two visceral areas that can refer to the lumbar spine are suggested; list any other sites or conditions you can think of, together with a simple way of deciding from where the symptoms are being referred.

Referral site / condition	How to determine from where the symptoms could be referred
Musculoskeletal referral	
Rheumatological condition	

Visceral referral
   Cardiovascular system
   (abdominal aorta)
 	
   Pelvic viscera	

The patient's age when the symptoms originally began may suggest specific underlying conditions. Using the following age groupings and headings, list what you consider these possible conditions may be.

0-20	Congenital	
	Developmental	
	Rheumatological	

20-40	Congenital	
	Developmental	
	Postural / occupational	
	Rheumatological	

40-60	Hormonal / age	
	Postural / occupational	
	Rheumatological	

60+	Degenerative	
	Hormonal / age	
	Rheumatological	

Generally, musculoskeletal symptoms occur following a specific event or gradually for no apparent reason over a period of days, months or years.

If the onset was sudden, resulting from one notable incident, suggest causes for the patient's symptoms bearing in mind your experience.

For the above indicate the primary tissues causing symptoms, together with your personal differential diagnostic rationale for selecting those tissues (aggravating and relieving features).

If the onset was for no apparent reason, suggest causes for the patient's symptoms bearing in mind your experience.

For the above indicate the primary tissues causing symptoms, together with your personal differential diagnostic rationale for selecting those tissues (aggravating and relieving features).

Indicate what spinal changes or named pathological conditions could occur in the lumbar spine of a postmenopausal woman or elderly male patient.

Continuing Professional Development
Record Sheet

To assist when submitting your CPD summary or for your portfolio, please use this page to identify the time spent working through this section.

Hands On: developing your differential diagnostic skills.

Name: ……………………………………………………………………………….. CPD year: ……................……

Date	Pages covered	Number of CPD hours		Venue / people involved
		Learning by oneself	Learning with others	

Date	Area	Identified areas for further study		Venue / people involved
		Learning by oneself	Learning with others	

Signature: …………………………................………… Date: …………..............

2.4.5 *Pelvis*

The pelvis refers to the synovial sacroiliac joints, the sacrococcygeal ligament and the fibrous symphysis pubis.

When taking a case history, it is important to remember that the symptoms can be originating from the pelvis, associated with another part of the musculoskeletal system, related to a rheumatological condition or referred from one of the body's other systems.

In the following box identify from where the pain or symptoms could be referred. One musculoskeletal area and two visceral areas that can refer to the pelvis are suggested; list any other sites or conditions you can think of, together with a simple way of deciding from where the symptoms are being referred.

Referral site / condition	How to determine from where the symptoms could be referred
Musculoskeletal referral Lumbar spine	
Rheumatological condition	
Visceral referral Pelvic viscera	
Abdominal viscera	

The patient's age when the symptoms originally began may suggest specific underlying conditions. Using the following age groupings and headings, list what you consider these possible conditions may be.

0-20	Congenital	
	Developmental	
	Rheumatological	

20-40	Congenital	
	Developmental	
	Postural / occupational	
	Rheumatological	

40-60	Hormonal / age	
	Postural / occupational	
	Rheumatological	

60+	Degenerative	
	Hormonal / age	
	Rheumatological	

Generally, musculoskeletal symptoms occur following a specific event or gradually for no apparent reason over a period of days, months or years.

If the onset was sudden, resulting from one notable incident, suggest causes for the patient's symptoms bearing in mind your experience.

Sacroiliac	
Sacrococcygeal	
Symphysis pubis	

For the above indicate the primary tissues causing symptoms, together with your personal differential diagnostic rationale for selecting those tissues (aggravating and relieving features). Identify which joint(s) the condition will affect.

Sacroiliac	
Sacrococcygeal	
Symphysis pubis	

If the onset was for no apparent reason, suggest causes for the patient's symptoms bearing in mind your experience.

Sacroiliac	
Sacrococcygeal	
Symphysis pubis	

For the above indicate the primary tissues causing symptoms, together with your personal differential diagnostic rationale for selecting those tissues (aggravating and relieving features). Identify which joint(s) the condition will affect.

Sacroiliac	
Sacrococcygeal	
Symphysis pubis	

2.4.6 Shoulder complex

The shoulder complex refers to the following synovial joints: glenohumeral, acromioclavicular and sternoclavicular, and the muscular scapulothoracic joint.

When taking a case history, it is important to remember that the symptoms can be originating from the shoulder complex, associated with another part of the musculoskeletal system, related to a rheumatological condition or referred from one of the body's other systems.

In the following box identify from where the pain or symptoms could be referred. One musculoskeletal area and several visceral areas that can refer to the shoulder complex are suggested; list any other sites or conditions you can think of, together with a simple way of deciding from where the symptoms are being referred.

Referral site / condition	How to determine from where the symptoms could be referred
Musculoskeletal referral Cervical spine	
Rheumatological condition	

Visceral referral
  Cardiovascular system
  (left or right shoulder)	

Respiratory system (diaphragm [left or right shoulder])	
Biliary system (right shoulder)	
Other (left shoulder)	

2.4.6 Shoulder complex

The patient's age when the symptoms originally began may suggest specific underlying conditions. Using the following age groupings and headings, list what you consider these possible conditions may be.

0-20
Congenital

Developmental

Rheumatological

20-40
Congenital

Developmental

Postural / occupational

Rheumatological

40-60
Hormonal / age

Postural / occupational

Rheumatological

60+
Degenerative

Hormonal / age

Rheumatological

Generally, musculoskeletal symptoms occur following a specific event or gradually for no apparent reason over a period of days, months or years.

If the onset was sudden, resulting from one notable incident, suggest causes for the patient's symptoms bearing in mind your experience.

For the above indicate the primary tissues causing symptoms, together with your personal differential diagnostic rationale for selecting those tissues (aggravating and relieving features).

If the onset was for no apparent reason, suggest causes for the patient's symptoms bearing in mind your experience.

For the above indicate the primary tissues causing symptoms, together with your personal differential diagnostic rationale for selecting those tissues (aggravating and relieving features).

2.4.7 Elbow joint complex

The elbow joint complex refers to the following synovial joints: humero-ulnar, humeroradial and superior radio-ulnar.

When taking a case history, it is important to remember that the symptoms can be originating from the elbow joint complex, associated with another part of the musculoskeletal system, related to a rheumatological condition or referred from one of the body's other systems.

In the following box identify from where the pain or symptoms could be referred. One musculoskeletal area that can refer to the elbow complex is suggested; list any other sites or conditions you can think of, together with a simple way of deciding from where the symptoms are being referred.

Referral site / condition	How to determine from where the symptoms could be referred
Musculoskeletal referral Cervical spine	
Rheumatological condition	
Visceral referral	

The patient's age when the symptoms originally began may suggest specific underlying conditions. Using the following age groupings and headings, list what you consider these possible conditions may be.

0-20	Congenital	
	Developmental	
	Rheumatological	

20-40	Congenital	
	Developmental	
	Postural / occupational	
	Rheumatological	

40-60	Hormonal / age	
	Postural / occupational	
	Rheumatological	

60+	Degenerative	
	Hormonal / age	
	Rheumatological	

Generally, musculoskeletal symptoms occur following a specific event or gradually for no apparent reason over a period of days, months or years.

If the onset was sudden, resulting from one notable incident, suggest causes for the patient's symptoms bearing in mind your experience.

For the above indicate the primary tissues causing symptoms, together with your personal differential diagnostic rationale for selecting those tissues (aggravating and relieving features).

2.4.7 Elbow joint complex

If the onset was for no apparent reason, suggest causes for the patient's symptoms bearing in mind your experience.

For the above indicate the primary tissues causing symptoms, together with your personal differential diagnostic rationale for selecting those tissues (aggravating and relieving features).

There are three named nerves that can be compressed at various sites round the elbow. Name the nerve affected, the tissue causing the compression and area of the resultant neurological symptoms.

2.4.8 Wrist and hand complex

The wrist complex refers to the distal radio-ulnar, carpal and metacarpal joints.

When taking a case history, it is important to remember that the symptoms can be originating from the wrist and hand complex, associated with another part of the musculoskeletal system, related to a rheumatological condition or referred from one of the body's other systems.

In the following box identify from where the pain or symptoms could be referred. Three visceral areas that can refer to the wrist and hand complex are suggested; list any other sites or conditions you can think of, together with a simple way of deciding from where the symptoms are being referred.

Referral site / condition	How to determine from where the symptoms could be referred
Musculoskeletal referral	
Rheumatological condition	
Visceral referral Cardiovascular system	
Respiratory system	
Endocrine system	

2.4.8 Wrist and hand complex

The patient's age when the symptoms originally began may suggest specific underlying conditions. Using the following age groupings and headings, list what you consider these possible conditions may be.

0-20	Congenital	
	Developmental	
	Rheumatological	

20-40	Congenital	
	Developmental	
	Postural / occupational	
	Rheumatological	

40-60	Hormonal / age	
	Postural / occupational	
	Rheumatological	

60+	Degenerative	
	Hormonal / age	
	Rheumatological	

Generally, musculoskeletal symptoms occur following a specific event or gradually for no apparent reason over a period of days, months or years.

If the onset was sudden, resulting from one notable incident, suggest causes for the patient's symptoms bearing in mind your experience.

For the above indicate the primary tissues causing symptoms, together with your personal differential diagnostic rationale for selecting those tissues (aggravating and relieving features).

If the onset was for no apparent reason, suggest causes for the patient's symptoms bearing in mind your experience.

For the above indicate the primary tissues causing symptoms, together with your personal differential diagnostic rationale for selecting those tissues (aggravating and relieving features).

What obvious deformities can develop in the wrist and hand?

Name the following deformities noting the common causes in each case.

Rheumatological / connective tissue   **Neurological**

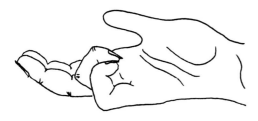

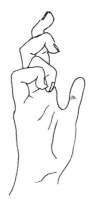

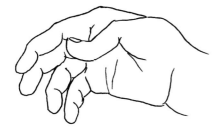

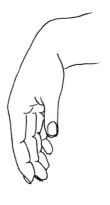

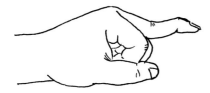

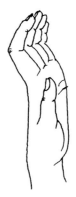

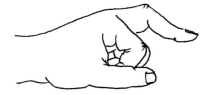

Figure 2.1 Deformities in the hand and wrist.

Continuing Professional Development Record Sheet

To assist when submitting your CPD summary or for your portfolio, please use this page to identify the time spent working through this section.

Hands On: developing your differential diagnostic skills.

Name: ………….. CPD year: …….................……

Date	Pages covered	Number of CPD hours		Venue / people involved
		Learning by oneself	Learning with others	

Date	Area	Identified areas for further study		Venue / people involved
		Learning by oneself	Learning with others	

Signature: …………………….....……………… Date: ……….............

2.4.9 Hip joint

When taking a case history, it is important to remember that the symptoms can be originating from the hip joint, associated with another part of the musculoskeletal system, related to a rheumatological condition or referred from one of the body's other systems.

In the following box identify from where the pain or symptoms could be referred. One musculoskeletal area and two visceral areas that can refer to the hip joint are suggested; list any other sites or conditions you can think of, together with a simple way of deciding from where the symptoms are being referred.

Referral site / condition	How to determine from where the symptoms could be referred
Musculoskeletal referral Psoas spasm	
Rheumatological condition	
Visceral referral Respiratory system	
Abdominal viscera	

The patient's age when the symptoms originally began will, particularly in the hip joint, suggest a specific underlying condition. Using the following age groupings and headings, list what you consider these possible conditions may be.

0-20	Congenital	
	Developmental	
	Rheumatological	

20-40	Congenital	
	Developmental	
	Postural / occupational	
	Rheumatological	

40-60	Hormonal / age	
	Postural / occupational	
	Rheumatological	

60+	Degenerative	
	Hormonal / age	
	Rheumatological	

Generally, musculoskeletal symptoms occur following a specific event or gradually for no apparent reason over a period of days, months or years.

If the onset was sudden, resulting from one notable incident, suggest causes for the patient's symptoms bearing in mind your experience.

2.4.9 Hip joint

For the above indicate the primary tissues causing symptoms, together with your personal differential diagnostic rationale for selecting those tissues (aggravating and relieving features).

If the onset was for no apparent reason, suggest causes for the patient's symptoms bearing in mind your experience.

For the above indicate the primary tissues causing symptoms, together with your personal differential diagnostic rationale for selecting those tissues (aggravating and relieving features).

2.4.10 Knee joint

The knee joint refers to the following synovial joints: tibiofemoral, patellofemoral and superior tibiofibular joints.

When taking a case history, it is important to remember that the symptoms can be originating from the knee joint, associated with another part of the musculoskeletal system, related to a rheumatological condition or referred from one of the body's other systems.

In the following box identify from where the pain or symptoms could be referred. One musculoskeletal area that can refer to the knee joint is suggested; list any other sites or conditions you can think of, together with a simple way of deciding from where the symptoms are being referred.

Referral site / condition	How to determine from where the symptoms could be referred
Musculoskeletal referral Hip joint	
Rheumatological condition	
Visceral referral	

2.4.10 Knee joint

The patient's age when the symptoms originally began may suggest specific underlying conditions. Using the following age groupings and headings, list what you consider these possible conditions may be.

0-20	Congenital	
	Developmental	
	Rheumatological	

20-40	Congenital	
	Developmental	
	Postural / occupational	
	Rheumatological	

40-60	Hormonal / age	
	Postural / occupational	
	Rheumatological	

60+	Degenerative	
	Hormonal / age	
	Rheumatological	

Generally, musculoskeletal symptoms occur following a specific event or gradually for no apparent reason over a period of days, months or years.

If the onset was sudden, resulting from one notable incident, suggest causes for the patient's symptoms bearing in mind your experience.

2.4.10 Knee joint

For the above indicate the primary tissues causing symptoms, together with your personal differential diagnostic rationale for selecting those tissues (aggravating and relieving features).

If the onset was for no apparent reason, suggest causes for the patient's symptoms bearing in mind your experience.

For the above indicate the primary tissues causing symptoms, together with your personal differential diagnostic rationale for selecting those tissues (aggravating and relieving features).

2.4.11 Ankle and foot complex

The ankle and foot complex refers to all the joints distal to the talocrural joint.

When taking a case history, it is important to remember that the symptoms can be originating from the ankle, or foot, associated with another part of the musculoskeletal system, related to a rheumatological condition or referred from one of the body's other systems.

In the following box identify from where the pain or symptoms could be referred. One visceral area that can refer to the ankle and foot complex is suggested; list any other sites or conditions you can think of, together with a simple way of deciding from where the symptoms are being referred.

Referral site / condition	How to determine from where the symptoms could be referred
Musculoskeletal referral	
Rheumatological condition	
Visceral referral Abdominal viscera	

The ankle and foot complex is one of the few areas in the body where the actual site of pain or symptoms can be of great assistance when reaching a differential diagnosis. Figure 2.2 is a representation of the rearfoot and ankle; Figure 2.3 represents the sole of the foot. On the following outline drawings indicate where the following conditions are classically felt. Add any other conditions you are aware of.

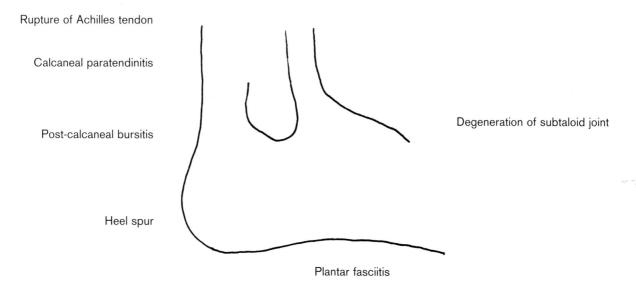

Rupture of Achilles tendon

Calcaneal paratendinitis

Post-calcaneal bursitis

Degeneration of subtaloid joint

Heel spur

Plantar fasciitis

Figure 2.2 Medial aspect of the ankle and rear foot.

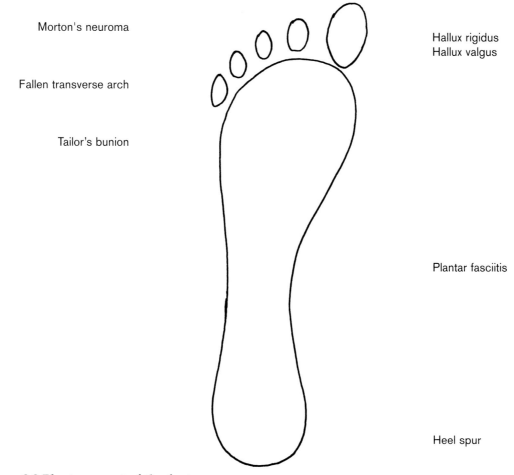

Morton's neuroma

Fallen transverse arch

Tailor's bunion

Hallux rigidus
Hallux valgus

Plantar fasciitis

Heel spur

Figure 2.3 Plantar aspect of the foot.

The patient's age when the symptoms originally began may suggest specific underlying conditions. Using the following age groupings and headings, list what you consider these possible conditions may be.

0-20	Congenital	
	Developmental	
	Rheumatological	

20-40	Congenital	
	Developmental	
	Postural / occupational	
	Rheumatological	

40-60	Hormonal / age	
	Postural / occupational	
	Rheumatological	

60+	Degenerative	
	Hormonal / age	
	Rheumatological	

2.4.11 Ankle and foot complex

The foot is considered in relation to its three functional areas: the rearfoot and ankle, the midfoot and the forefoot.

Generally, musculoskeletal symptoms occur following a specific event or gradually for no apparent reason over a period of days, months or years.

If the onset was sudden, resulting from one notable incident, suggest causes for the patient's symptoms bearing in mind your experience.

Rearfoot and ankle	Midfoot	Forefoot

For the above indicate the primary tissues causing symptoms, together with your personal differential diagnostic rationale for selecting those tissues (aggravating and relieving features).

Rearfoot and ankle	Midfoot	Forefoot

If the onset was for no apparent reason, suggest causes for the patient's symptoms bearing in mind your experience.

Rearfoot and ankle	Midfoot	Forefoot

For the above indicate the primary tissues causing symptoms, together with your personal differential diagnostic rationale for selecting those tissues (aggravating and relieving features).

Rearfoot and ankle	Midfoot	Forefoot

Continuing Professional Development
Record Sheet

To assist when submitting your CPD summary or for your portfolio, please use this page to identify the time spent working through this section.

Hands On: developing your differential diagnostic skills.

Name: ……………………………………………………………………………………… CPD year: ………………………

| Date | Pages covered | Number of CPD hours | | Venue / people involved |
		Learning by oneself	Learning with others	

| Date | Area | Identified areas for further study | | Venue / people involved |
		Learning by oneself	Learning with others	

Signature: ……………………………………… Date: ………………………

2.5 General health indicators and issues

Once the initial musculoskeletal complaint has been recorded, the patient's medical history is investigated, initially by asking about general health and health indicators (height, weight, current and previous medication) and later by questions directed at specific systemic systems.

In the next box some common indicators for general health are listed; suggest what underlying systemic condition(s) could be associated with these indicators.

General health indicator	Underlying condition suggested

Weight
    Unexpected weight gain
    Unexpected weight loss	

General health
    Fair
    Poor
    Always getting colds/flu	

Height Sudden loss of height	

Alcohol
    Female 14+ units per week
    Male 21+ units per week	

Smoking	
Recreational drugs	
Sensitivity to hot / cold	

In the previous box various general health indicators are listed. List any other questions regarding their general health, or perception of general health that you would ask the patient. Indicate what aspects of their general health they are designed to investigate: physical and psychosocial.

Endocrine dysfunction can often become apparent when asking general questions of the patient's general health, as the symptoms often develop slowly with the patient and close family oblivious to the problem. Without our intervention these conditions may only be identified when advanced, or when distant family or friends notice changes (physical or mental) in the patient.

Whilst taking the case history, careful observation of the patient may suggest an endocrine problem. In the following box three signs have been listed; specify why these indicate possible underlying endocrine disease. Can you think of any other signs of an endocrine disorder that could be apparent just by looking at the patient?

Specific sign or predictor	Linked endocrine problem
Exceptionally large hands	
Size of neck	
Tremor	
Other signs	

There are several musculoskeletal conditions that can be associated with disorders of the endocrine system. In the following box identify the associated endocrine problems.

Condition	Linked endocrine problem
Carpal tunnel syndrome	
Osteoporosis	
Muscle or bone pain	
Other conditions	

2.5 General health indicators

Two common endocrine problems that may become apparent when considering the patient's general health are related to insulin and thyroxine production. In the following three boxes list the common signs associated with abnormal production of these two hormones that may be identified when discussing the patient's general health.

Insulin and diabetes (type 2)

Thyroxine and hypothyroidism

Thyroxine and hyperthyroidism

General signs or symptoms of endocrine dysfunction can be elicited when considering symptoms from other bodily systems. Indicate what general symptoms from the named systems would suggest a possible endocrine dysfunction or disease was present, and suggest why.

System	Symptoms	Linked endocrine problem
Cardiovascular		
Respiratory		
Gastrointestinal		
Neurological		
Urinary		
Reproductive		

Continuing Professional Development Record Sheet

To assist when submitting your CPD summary or for your portfolio, please use this page to identify the time spent working through this section.

Hands On: developing your differential diagnostic skills.

Name: ……………………………………………………………………………… CPD year: ………................……

Date	Pages covered	Number of CPD hours		Venue / people involved
		Learning by oneself	**Learning with others**	

Date	Area	Identified areas for further study		Venue / people involved
		Learning by oneself	**Learning with others**	

Signature: ……………………………….......……………… Date: ………...............

2.6 Past medical history indicators and issues

The past medical history will give vital information about the general state of the patient's health and medical wellbeing, and identifying pre-existing conditions will enable the practitioner to decide the most suitable form of treatment. In the following section each of the main bodily systems are covered in turn. Identify what questions you would initially ask to investigate the signs and symptoms of the common conditions associated with each system, and indicate how the presence of these conditions would modify your general treatment plan.

2.6.1 Cardiovascular system

When questioning a patient about a specific system, the first priority is to ask the right questions. It is important to ask a general question first, followed by more specific questions.

The general question could be:

♦   'Have you ever suffered with heart / circulatory problems in the past?'
    If the answer is **no**, the next question could be:
♦   'Have you ever suffered from _____?' (note in the box below three different questions that may uncover an underlying cardiovascular condition. Remember to use simple terms that the patient will understand).

1)
2)
3)

If the answer to the general question above was **yes**, note in the following box common cardiovascular disorders and associated symptoms you would expect the patient to mention.

Common cardiovascular conditions	Associated symptoms

In a very general way use the following box to indicate how these identified common cardiovascular conditions might affect a patient's posture, activities or lifestyle. Speculate how these changes may generate musculoskeletal symptoms and suggest a very general treatment plan (aims and objectives) that would assist this patient.

2.6.2 Respiratory system

When questioning a patient about a specific system, the first priority is to ask the right questions. It is important to ask a general question first, followed by more specific questions.

The general question could be:

♦ 'Have you ever suffered with chest / breathing problems in the past?'
  If the answer is **no**, the next question could be:
♦ 'Have you ever suffered from _____ ?' (note in the box below three different questions that may uncover an underlying respiratory condition. Remember to use simple terms that the patient will understand).

1)
2)
3)

If the answer to the general question above was **yes**, then note in the following box common respiratory disorders and the associated symptoms you would expect the patient to mention.

Common respiratory conditions	Associated symptoms

In a very general way use the following box to indicate how these identified common respiratory conditions might affect a patient's posture, activities or lifestyle. Speculate how these changes may generate musculoskeletal symptoms and suggest a very general treatment plan (aims and objectives) that would assist this patient.

2.6.3 Gastrointestinal system

When questioning a patient about a specific system, the first priority is to ask the right questions. It is important to ask a general question first, followed by more specific questions.

The general question could be:

♦ 'Have you ever suffered with digestive problems in the past?'
  If the answer is **no**, the next question could be
♦ 'Have you ever suffered from   ?' (note in the box below three different questions that may uncover an underlying gastrointestinal condition. Remember to use simple terms that the patient will understand).

1)
2)
3)

If the answer to the general question above was **yes**, then note in the following box common gastrointestinal disorders and the associated symptoms you would expect the patient to mention.

Common gastrointestinal conditions	Associated symptoms

In a very general way use the following box to indicate how these identified common digestive conditions might affect a patient's posture, activities or lifestyle. Speculate how these changes may generate musculoskeletal symptoms and suggest a very general treatment plan (aims and objectives) that would assist this patient.

Continuing Professional Development Record Sheet

To assist when submitting your CPD summary or for your portfolio, please use this page to identify the time spent working through this section.

Hands On: developing your differential diagnostic skills.

Name: .... CPD year: ....

| Date | Pages covered | Number of CPD hours | | Venue / people involved |
		Learning by oneself	Learning with others	

| Date | Area | Identified areas for further study | | Venue / people involved |
		Learning by oneself	Learning with others	

Signature: .... Date: ....

2.6.4 Neurological system

When questioning a patient about a specific system, the first priority is to ask the right questions. It is important to ask a general question first, followed by more specific questions.

The general question could be:

- 'Have you ever suffered with neurological problems in the past?'
  If the answer is **no**, the next question could be
- 'Have you ever suffered from _____?' (note in the box below three different questions that may uncover an underlying neurological condition. Remember to use simple terms that the patient will understand).

1)
2)
3)

If the answer to the general question above was **yes**, then note in the following box common neurological disorders and the associated symptoms you would expect the patient to mention.

Common neurological conditions	Associated symptoms

In a very general way use the following box to indicate how these identified common neurological conditions might affect a patient's posture, activities or lifestyle. Speculate how these changes may generate musculoskeletal symptoms and suggest a very general treatment plan (aims and objectives) that would assist this patient.

2.6.5 *Urinary and reproductive systems*

When questioning a patient about a specific system, the first priority is to ask the right questions. It is important to ask a general question first, followed by more specific questions. In the box below construct a suitable question for each of the two systems. Remember to use simple words and non-medical terms that will not embarrass the patient.

Urinary system

Reproductive / gynaecological system

If the answer is **no**, the next question could be:

♦ 'Have you ever suffered from   ? ' (note in the box below two simple questions that could be asked to identify the presence of an underlying urinary [not prostate] or reproductive disorder. Remember to use simple terms that the patient will understand).

1)

2)

In the next box write down a general question that would, without embarrassment to the patient, give you an indication of the degree of any prostatic hypertrophy present.

If the answer to the general question, 'Have you ever suffered with urinary or gynaecological problems in the past?' was **yes**, then note in the following two boxes common urinary or gynaecological disorders and the associated symptoms you would expect the patient to mention.

Common urinary conditions	Associated symptoms

Common gynaecological conditions	Associated symptoms

In a very general way use the following box to indicate how these identified common conditions might affect a patient's posture, activities or lifestyle. Speculate how these changes may generate musculoskeletal symptoms and suggest a very general treatment plan (aims and objectives) that would assist this patient.

2.6.6 Ear, nose and throat

When questioning a patient about a specific system, the first priority is to ask the right questions. It is important to ask a general question first, followed by more specific questions.

The general question could be:

♦ 'Have you ever suffered with ear, nose and throat problems in the past?'
   If the answer is **no**, the next question could be:

♦ 'Have you ever suffered from _____?' (note in the box below one simple question for each area that might uncover an underlying ear, nose and throat condition. Remember to use simple terms that the patient will understand).

Ear
Nose
Throat

If the answer to the general question above was **yes**, then note in the following three boxes common ear, nose and throat disorders and the associated symptoms you would expect the patient to mention.

Common ear problems	Associated symptoms

Common nose problems	Associated symptoms

Common throat problems	Associated symptoms

In a very general way use the following box to indicate how these identified common ear, nose or throat conditions might affect a patient's posture, activities or lifestyle. Speculate how these changes may generate musculoskeletal symptoms and suggest a very general treatment plan (aims and objectives) that would assist this patient.

Continuing Professional Development
Record Sheet

To assist when submitting your CPD summary or for your portfolio, please use this page to identify the time spent working through this section.

Hands On: developing your differential diagnostic skills.

Name: ………………………………………………………………………… CPD year: …………...........……

Date	Pages covered	Number of CPD hours		Venue / people involved
		Learning by oneself	Learning with others	

Date	Area	Identified areas for further study		Venue / people involved
		Learning by oneself	Learning with others	

Signature: …………………………......…………… Date: ………….............

Evaluation

3.1 Observation

Once the patient is stripped to their underwear and you begin the normal physical evaluation, many signs, often of systemic disease, can be observed, from varicose veins to surgical scars. On Figure 3.1 indicate where you would expect to see scars for the named operations.

Appendix   Caesarean   Carpal tunnel   Gall bladder
Heart   Hip replacement   Hysterectomy   Knee cartilage
Kidney   Laparoscopy   Lumbar disc   Varicose veins

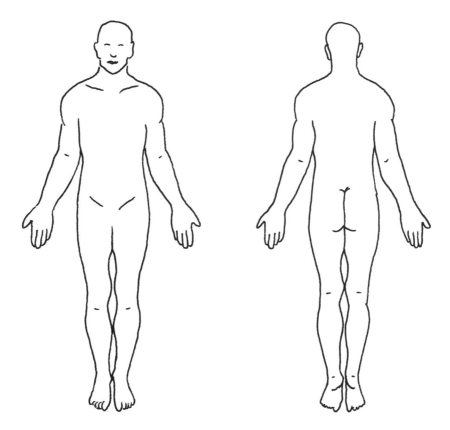

Figure 3.1 Outline of the body: anterior and posterior.

In the following box are various non-specific signs you would probably notice whilst observing the patient. What do they suggest to you?

Signs	Suggesting
Male wearing incontinence pants	
Obvious urine stains on underwear	
Female wearing panty liners	
Blood on underwear	

What could the following dermatological signs indicate to the observant practitioner?

Multiple scars on the forearms

A dirty brown discoloration to the ankles and feet

A yellowish tinge to the skin

The patient suffers with psoriasis. How is this observed skin complaint related to joint pain?

Are there any other dermatological signs that may suggest an underlying systemic or musculoskeletal condition?

Whilst generally observing the patient, a note of the depth, rate and rhythm of respiration can be made. What observations would suggest that a respiratory or cardiovascular examination is necessary?

Specific signs of systemic disease tend to be apparent in specific sites, generally in the skin and particularly in the skin of the hands, feet and abdomen. In the following box indicate what signs can be apparent in these areas and what underlying system they incriminate.

Site	Signs	System(s) incriminated
Skin General		
Abdomen / thorax		
Hands / fingers		
Feet / ankles		

Dysfunction of the endocrine system will give generalised signs that can be observed. What particular endocrine conditions do the following clinical signs suggest?

Aspect	Feature	Endocrine condition
Skin	Scar (colour)	
	Excessive / minimal perspiration	
Hair (changes from normal)	Greasy / very dry	
Nails (changes from normal)	Fragile	

3.2 Palpation

Most information relating to systemic disease would be identified from the case history initially and then confirmed by a specific systemic examination routine. Where a specific systemic examination routine has not been indicated, what general signs of systemic disease could be identified from palpation? In the following box two common findings from palpation have been identified. Which systems would these findings incriminate and why?

General sign	System	Reason
Temperature Very localised change		
Regional change		
General increase / decrease		
Oedema Pitting		
Non-pitting		
Other signs		

Continuing Professional Development
Record Sheet

To assist when submitting your CPD summary or for your portfolio, please use this page to identify the time spent working through this section.

Hands On: developing your differential diagnostic skills.

Name: ………...……… CPD year: ……...............……

Date	Pages covered	Number of CPD hours		Venue / people involved
		Learning by oneself	Learning with others	

Date	Area	Identified areas for further study		Venue / people involved
		Learning by oneself	Learning with others	

Signature: …………………......…………. Date: ……….............

Section 4

Specific system examination

Throughout this section it will be assumed that you are competent and well practised in specific system examination procedures. This section will therefore concentrate upon what might be considered to be abnormal findings and exploring your clinical diagnostic skills when presented with these changes from the normal.

4.1 Cardiovascular system examination

During your observation and palpation of the patient you are alert to specific signs of cardiovascular disease. In the following box briefly list these signs.

4.1.1 Auscultation

When conducting auscultation of the heart, it is noticed that the apex beat is not in the 5th intercostal space in the mid-clavicular line. What medical conditions could cause this change in position?

What structural conditions may cause the same finding?

4.1.2 Percussion

In the following box indicate what information you gain from percussing the heart.

When completing a cardiovascular examination, the abdomen can be palpated and percussed. In the following box answer the questions relating to examination of the abdomen during a cardiovascular examination.

Why is the abdomen palpated?

What palpatory findings would indicate an abnormality?

Why is the abdomen percussed?

What findings would indicate an abnormality?

4.1.3 Measurement of blood pressure

This is a very common and simple procedure to undertake that, it could be argued, should be conducted on every patient. What are the arguments, both for and against, this point of view?

In the clinical environment, problems arise, equipment is forgotten or broken.

How can you make an assessment of a patient's systolic blood pressure if your stethoscope is missing?

How can you make an assessment of a patient's blood pressure if your sphygmomanometer is broken?

4.2 Respiratory system examination

During your observation and palpation of the patient, you are alert to specific signs of respiratory disease. In the following box briefly list these signs.

4.2.1 Auscultation

In the following box outline what the following terms for breath sounds indicate and describe the sound.

Adventitious breath sounds
(description)

Discontinuous breath sounds
(description)

Continuous breath sounds
(description)

Lack of breath sounds
(description)

Normal voice sounds are muffled and indistinct. In the following box indicate what could cause them to be enhanced or absent.

Voice sounds enhanced because
Voice sounds absent because

4.2.2 Percussion

When percussing the thorax, different sounds or resonance will indicate different underlying problems. In the following box indicate what the identified sound suggests regarding the lung tissue.

Sound	Underlying condition
Flatness	
Dullness	
Resonance	
Hyper-resonance	
Tympany	

4.3 Gastrointestinal system examination

During your observation and palpation of the patient you are alert to specific signs of gastrointestinal disease. In the following box briefly list these signs.

4.3.1 Auscultation

When conducting auscultation of the abdomen, the normal borborygmi can be heard every 10 seconds. In the box some additional sounds that can be heard are noted. List the various causes of these sounds and add any other sounds, together with their causes.

Noise heard	Causes
No sound	
Fluid 'sploshing' around	
Hyper-resonance	
Peritoneal rub	
Other sounds	

4.3.2 Percussion

In the following box answer these two questions relating to percussion of the abdomen.

What important structures can you identify when percussing the abdomen?

In addition to air, what features / conditions can you identify when percussing the abdomen?

4.3.3 *Palpation*

Palpation is a vital tool when trying to identify abdominal structures. In the following box explain why palpation should begin away from any identified tender areas.

In the following box list the organs / structures identified by light or deep palpation.

Light palpation

Deep palpation

In the following box answer the following questions.

Name the vital pulsating structure that should always be palpated in the abdomen.

Where is the pulsation palpated in relation to the umbilicus?

In which direction is the pulsation normally detected (anteriorly or laterally)?

What clinical emergency may be suggested if the pulsation is increased or displaced laterally?

Continuing Professional Development Record Sheet

To assist when submitting your CPD summary or for your portfolio, please use this page to identify the time spent working through this section.

Hands On: developing your differential diagnostic skills.

Name: ……………………………………………………………………………………………….. CPD year: ………..............……

Date	Pages covered	Number of CPD hours		Venue / people involved
		Learning by oneself	Learning with others	

Date	Area	Identified areas for further study		Venue / people involved
		Learning by oneself	Learning with others	

Signature: ……………………………......…………… Date: ……….............

4.4 Neurological system examination

When undertaking a neurological examination, it is important to remember to examine the peripheral nerves, and whenever necessary, to be able to check for abnormal function of the cranial nerves.

Signs of neurological deficit can be generally described as motor (altered muscular function) or sensory (altered skin sensation or joint proprioception).

During your observation of the patient you are alert to specific signs of neurological disease. In the following box briefly list these signs.

4.4.1 Palpation

In the following box indicate the general changes palpated in the named neurological conditions.

Are there any other neurological conditions that should be included in this box?

Neurological conditions	Muscle tone	Sensory signs
Multiple sclerosis		
Peripheral neuropathy		
Bell's palsy		
Cerebrovascular accident		
Peripheral nerve lesion		
Parkinson's disease		
Other diseases		

4.4.2 Sensory neurological examination

A sensory neurological loss will have an obvious effect upon how the patient perceives external stimuli. In the following box describe your routine for identifying the extent of sensory loss and how you would test for it.

In the following box state what the loss of vibration sense, light touch or pinprick indicates.

Loss	Indicating
Vibration sense	
Light touch	
Pinprick	

Whenever the sensory aspect of the neurological system is affected, there will be an alteration in the patient's perception of touch or joint position. In the following box several neurological conditions that can affect sensation or joint positional sense have been listed. Indicate what the palpation findings (area of sensory loss) would be in each case, suggesting how it would be tested. Are there any other nerve diseases that should be included in this box?

Condition	Area of sensory / joint positional loss	How tested
Nerve root lesion		
Peripheral nerve lesion		
Diabetic neuropathy		
Dorsal column lesion		
Cerebrovascular accident		
Other conditions		

Figure 4.1 indicates the anterior and posterior dermal distribution of the spinal nerve roots to the upper and lower extremity. Identify and label the nerve root that supplies the areas demarcated by the dotted lines.

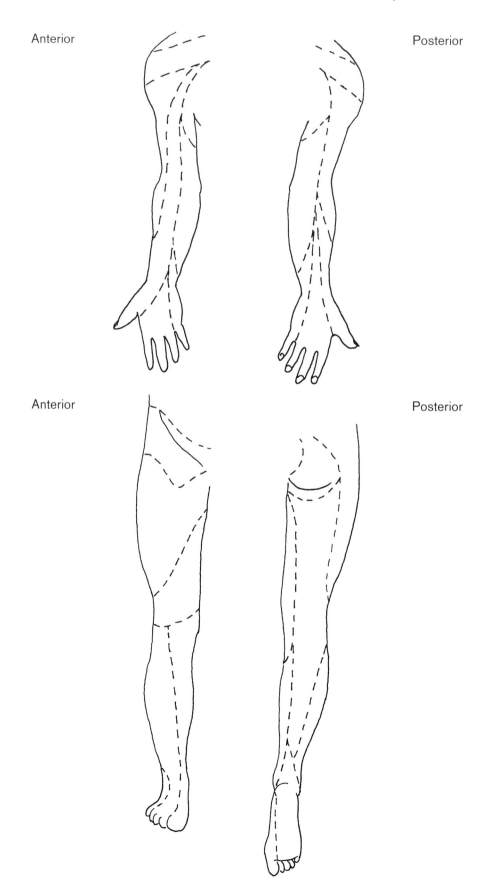

Anterior

Posterior

Anterior

Posterior

Figure 4.1 Anterior and posterior dermal distribution of the spinal nerve root.

Figure 4.2 indicates the anterior and posterior dermal distribution of the peripheral nerves to the upper and lower extremity. Identify the peripheral nerves that supply the areas demarcated by the dotted lines.

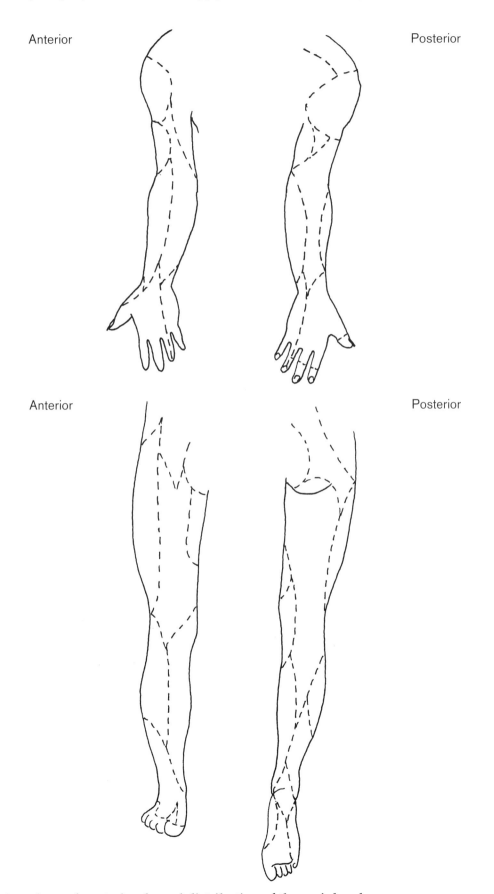

Anterior

Posterior

Anterior

Posterior

Figure 4.2 Anterior and posterior dermal distribution of the peripheral nerves.

4.4.3 Motor neurological examination

The testing of reflexes are regularly carried out in the consulting room. Briefly describe how the deep muscular reflex works.

When testing reflexes note which specific nerve root(s) is / are being tested with the following deep muscular reflexes.

Maxillary	Patella
Biceps	Achilles
Triceps	
Brachioradialis (periosteoradial)	

Several reflexes disappear in childhood. Name and briefly describe these infantile reflexes.

Pathological reflexes are reflexes that are not normally present in the healthy patient. Indicate how the following pathological reflexes / signs are tested and what response would constitute an abnormal response.

Plantar reflex
Gordon's finger sign
Hoffmann's sign
McCarthy's sign

Assessing the power of muscles will assist in determining the level or type of neurological lesion.

If the neurological damage was in a specific peripheral nerve, what muscle power findings would be present?

If the neurological damage was in a specific spinal nerve root, what muscle power findings would be present?

If the neurological damage was in the spinal cord or above, what muscle power findings would be present?

4.4.3 Motor neurological examination

A quick screening test linking muscle weakness with individual spinal nerve roots compares the strength of different body movements. Identify the movements linked with each spinal nerve root.

Spinal level	Resisted movement	Spinal level	Resisted movement
C1		L2	
C2		L3	
C3		L4	
C4		L5	
C5		S1	
C6			
C7			
C8			
T1			

The cranial nerves arise directly from the brain and supply various structures of the head and neck. Each cranial nerve supplies specific areas or organs of the head and neck.

In the following box indicate how the cranial nerves could be tested and what the abnormal findings associated with each individual cranial nerve would be.

Cranial nerve	Test	Abnormal findings
I		
II		
III		
IV		
V		
VI		
VII		
VIII		
IX		
X		
XI		
XII		

When a full neurological examination has been completed, a combination of various signs will suggest either an upper or lower neurone problem is present. Indicate what response (increased or reduced; present or absent) would be considered a sign of a problem in the central (upper sign) and peripheral (lower sign) nervous system.

Upper sign		Lower sign
	Peripheral reflexes	
	Specific muscle weakness (single nerve supply)	
	Limb tremor	
	Muscle fasciculation	
	Impaired coordination / balance	
	General muscle weakness (multiple nerve supply)	
	Altered gait	
	Joint position sense	
	Involuntary resistance to joint movement	
	Pathological reflex present	
	Infantile reflex present in infant	
	Glove stocking paraesthesia / numbness	
	Infantile reflex present in child / adult	
	Dermatomal paraesthesia / numbness	
	Stereognosis / graphaesthesia	
	Vibration sense	

Continuing Professional Development
Record Sheet

To assist when submitting your CPD summary or for your portfolio, please use this page to identify the time spent working through this section.

Hands On: developing your differential diagnostic skills.

Name: ………………………………………………………………………………………… CPD year: ………................……

Date	Pages covered	Number of CPD hours		Venue / people involved
		Learning by oneself	Learning with others	

Date	Area	Identified areas for further study		Venue / people involved
		Learning by oneself	Learning with others	

Signature: ……………………………......………… Date: ……….............

Section 5

Sample answers

In this section sample answers are provided for questions posed throughout the workbook. The answers provided are intentionally brief, and as mentioned in the Introduction, should only be used as a **starting point** for further thought, research or reading after writing your first answer in the body of the workbook.

Further information can be found in *Hands On: A Clinical Companion. Steps to confidence in musculoskeletal diagnosis* (ISBN 1 903378 30 3; tfm publishing)

In this section each answer box is identified by page number and in some cases the original question is included. The format of the question box is the same as in the main body of the book.

Section 1 General observation of the patient
1.1 Musculoskeletal system
Page 1

Patient's age	Degenerative, congenital or developmental condition Rheumatological disorder Specific pathological disease process
Patient's gender	Hormonal condition Specific pathology Rheumatological condition
Patient's posture	Degree of pain / disability Specific joint problem
Accompanying support aids	Duration of problem Friends / family who need assistance (aid borrowed)

1.2 Systemic system
Page 2

Specific predictors	Which system(s) affected
Patient smokes	Respiratory, cardiovascular, reproductive

Specific signs	Which system(s) affected
Facial skin colour:	
yellowish hue	Liver problem
red/ruddy	Respiratory, cardiovascular
blue tinge to lips	Cardiovascular
Unsuitable clothing considering the ambient outside temperature	Hormonal, endocrine
Constant blowing of nose	Respiratory, autoimmune

1.3 Psychosocial issues

Page 3

The demeanour of the patient may give an insight to the degree of strain that they are under, and whether it has affected them in the short or long term. In the following box indicate what signs of psychological strain can be apparent. State if it is possible to determine if the signs are due to short- or long-term psychosocial issues.

Fingernails bitten: long-term

Angle of shoulders indicating tension: long-term

Seated posture indicating tension / pain: short or long-term

1.4 Other signs or predictors

Signs	Musculoskeletal system	Systemic systems
Breathlessness	Rib problem Poor physical fitness	Respiratory Cardiovascular
Difficulty in sitting	Pain avoidance	Cardiovascular (haemorrhoids) Psychiatric Dermatological

Page 4

Signs	Musculoskeletal system	Systemic systems
Altered gait	Pain avoidance Joint degeneration Rheumatological (rheumatoid arthritis) Skeletal deformity	Neurological (Parkinson's disease)
Poor mobility of specific joint(s)	Pain avoidance Localised joint problem Rheumatological (gout)	Neurological (muscular weakness)
Poor mobility in general	Pain avoidance Generalised degeneration Rheumatological (ankylosing spondylitis)	Neurological (multiple sclerosis, cerebrovascular accident)
Unsteadiness	Pain avoidance	Neurological (cerebrovascular accident) Inner ear Endocrine (diabetes affecting foot) Alcohol / drug abuse (prescription or recreational)

1.4 Other signs or predictors
2.1 General musculoskeletal signs

Section 2 Aspects of the case history process
2.1 General musculoskeletal signs and symptoms
Page 7

Acute pain	A recent onset or The degree of pain reflected by the degree of inflammation and physical tissue damage
Sub-acute pain	The degree of pain
Chronic pain	Long-standing pain or The degree of pain dramatically exceeding tissue damage (psychosocial overtones)

Page 8

Neurological pathways	Gate control theory (Melzach and Wall, modified and updated): will increase or decrease pain Dubrier (1997) - nervous tissue could alter sensitivity following tissue injury: will increase or reduce pain
Internal factors	Anxiety / stress / depression / pain behaviour - will increase pain Personal beliefs of pain / expectations - will increase or reduce pain
External factors	Heat / cold - will increase or reduce pain

Many patients suffer with chronic or recurrent conditions. What specific factors, physical and psychological, can modify the pain felt at the initial episode of the condition to that felt after many recurrences of the problem?

Physical factors:	modification of activities, added strain to local or distant structures causes disruption of tissues associated with the area causing original pain
Psychological factors:	pain can be modified by previous experience, tissue memory, expectations of the patient

Page 9

Congenital	From birth, or very young age, recurrent, progressively increasing frequency
Developmental	From mid to late teenage or early 20s, recurrent, progressively increasing frequency
Rheumatological	Pattern of pain, joint involvement, age of onset
Underlying neoplastic	Unremitting pain, night pain, weight loss
Referral from a specific system	Symptoms related to systems function
Degenerative	Age of patient, recurrent, progressively increasing intensity
Musculoskeletal	Symptoms related to specific area function

2.1.1 Local musculoskeletal tissue
Page 10

Tissue causing symptoms	Aggravating movements / activities	Relieving movements / activities
Muscle	Contraction of muscle	Rest, heat
Ligament	Stretch (end of range)	Gentle mobility
Facet / joint	Movement	Static
Disc	Weight / compression	Off weight-bearing
Bursa	Compression	Distraction
Fat pad	Compression	No compression
Bone	Weight, pressure	Support

Tissue / state	Modify symptoms by
Acute inflammation (<6 weeks)	Increased sensitivity of all tissues
Sub-acute inflammation	Intermittent pain, 'catches'
Chronic inflammation (>6 weeks)	Specific aggravating / relieving factors

2.1.2 *Rheumatological and systemic conditions*
Page 11

Indicators	A positive diagnosis in the past, joint deformities
General symptoms	Pattern of symptoms, associated systemic symptoms
General signs	Dermatological rash, joint deformities

A selection of the common rheumatological conditions, the typical joints affected and frequent systemic symptoms are listed.

Joint pain	Named rheumatological conditions	Joints affected	Systemic symptoms / signs
Monoarthritic pain	Gout	1st toe, occasionally ankle, knee, finger, single joint	Hypertension, renal stones
Symmetrical polyarthritic pain	Rheumatoid arthritis	Small joints: hands / feet; large joints: knees / shoulder	Lymphadenopathy, scleritis granulomatous lesions in myocardium, anaemia
	Systemic lupus erythematosus	Similar to RA. Small joints: hands / feet; large joints	Butterfly rash, pleurisy, heart murmurs, hypertension
	Polymyalgia rheumatica	Shoulder and / or pelvic girdle	Temporal arteritis
	Spondyloarthropathies	Pelvis progressively up spine	Iritis
Asymmetrical polyarthritic pain	Reiter's syndrome	Knee, ankle, foot; also, upper limb joints and spine	Urethritis, conjunctivitis
	Paget's disease	Hip, knee, lumbar and thoracic spine	None

Page 12

The commoner presenting signs and symptoms and the associated conditions that need to be excluded are listed.

'Syndrome'	Identifying symptoms or signs	Differential diagnosis
ME	Multiple pain areas	Rheumatoid arthritis, osteoarthritis, brain tumour
Fibromyalgia	Impaired memory	Neurological disease
	Rash / itches	Dermatitis, psoriasis, eczema
	Digestive disturbance	Crohn's disease, ulcerative colitis
	Eye irritation	Reiter's syndrome, infection
Irritable bowel syndrome (IBS)	Altered bowel habits	Rectal neoplasm, Crohn's disease, ulcerative colitis

A selection of the common conditions, the typical joints affected and frequent systemic symptoms are listed.

Joint pain	Named systemic conditions	Joints affected	Systemic symptoms / signs
Monoarthritic pain	Tuberculosis	Spine, hip, knee	Pain, night sweats, stiffness
	Lyme's disease	Large joints	Cranial nerve palsies, meningitis
	Endocarditis	Distal interphalangeal joint	Heart murmurs, splenomegaly

Page 13

Psoriasis can present with asymmetrical joint symptoms or when associated with a seronegative arthritis, symmetrical joint symptoms.

Joint pain	Named systemic conditions	Joints affected	Systemic symptoms / signs
Symmetrical polyarthritic pain	Psoriasis	Distal interphalangeal joint	Skin lesions, nail changes, iritis
Asymmetrical polyarthritic pain	Psoriasis	Distal interphalangeal joint	Skin lesions, nail changes, iritis
	Ulcerative colitis and Crohn's disease	Knees, ankles, occasionally other peripheral joints. It may be migratory	Abdominal pain, diarrhoea, weight loss, erythema nodosum, buccal ulceration

2.2 Predisposing and precipitating factors, physical and physiological
2.2.1 Physical factors
Short-term factors

Sitting posture (easy chair)

Physical activities: gardening, decorating, DIY activities out of the ordinary

Page 14
Long-term factors

Work posture

Sleeping posture (bed support)

Underlying muscular support, poor core stability

Condition	Precautions taken and why
Rheumatoid arthritis	Care with active and passive movement due to laxity of ligaments in the cervical spine, in particular the alar and cruciform ligaments of the atlas / axis
Marfan's syndrome	Care with active and passive movement due to generalised joint hypermobility
Down's syndrome	Care with active and passive movement due to ligament instability of the cervical spine
Turner's syndrome	Care to exclude associated endocrine and cervical problems
Graves' disease	Care to exclude associated hormonal conditions (hyperthyroidism)

Page 15

Long-term oral steroid therapy	Reduced 'normal' inflammatory response
	Reduced 'normal' immune response to infection
	Osteoporosis

2.2.2 Physiological factors

When the patient is faced with an emotionally stressful situation, what is the normal short-term physiological response to this 'stress' that occurs within their body?

Describe the effects of the response, from hypothalamus to end organ, listing the common signs or symptoms associated with this fight or flight reaction.

The hypothalamus stimulates the endocrine system and sympathetic nervous system

The endocrine system increases cortisol and aldosterone levels which in turn increases blood sugar levels, blood pressure and fluid retention. This reduces the immune response and inflammation

The sympathetic nervous system increases blood pressure, heart rate, blood sugar levels and reduces digestion

Page 16

Previously, the body's physiological response to the fight or flight reaction was described. If the stressful situation does not resolve quickly, how will the body's internal response be modified? In the following box describe how the response is physiologically modified and how this will affect any physical signs and symptoms. Indicate the possible long-term effects on the body of this altered physiological response.

Prolonged increase of cortisol production leads to:

hyperglycaemia, increased insulin production and possibly type 2 diabetes

suppression of the immune system

hypertension and arteriosclerosis

2.3 Symptoms referred from the systemic system
Page 17

In this box the common areas for symptom referral are noted together with an indication of the nature of symptoms. The aggravating and relieving factors will depend upon the specific underlying condition and those listed below are designed to give a brief overview of the typical symptom picture.

System	Referral to	Nature of symptoms	Aggravated by	Relieved by
Cardiovascular	Shoulders, arms, neck	Sharp crushing	Emotion, stress, activity	Rest, medication
Respiratory	Thorax	Breathless	Exercise exertion	Rest, inhaler, oxygen
Upper digestive tract	Retrosternal	Burning / flatulence	Flexion, relation to food	Sleeping propped up, medication
Small intestine	Variable abdomen	Variable altered stools	Specific foods	Specific food avoidance / types
Lower digestive tract	Pelvis	Altered bowel habit, flatus	Stress, food	Medication
Genitourinary	Pelvis	Burning on urination, discharge	Urination	-
Gynaecological	Low back and abdomen	Acute pain, aching, cramping	Monthly cycle	-
Biliary	Right shoulder	Bloating, acute colic pain	High fat diet	Low fat diet, surgery

Page 18

Condition	Systemic symptoms / signs	Joints affected	Joint pain pattern
Ulcerative colitis	Severe abdominal pains Relapses / remissions	Knees, ankles, often during remission	Asymmetrical
Crohn's disease	Variable and depends on the part of colon affected	Knees, ankles	Asymmetrical
IBS	Colicky, cramping, bloating	Similar to chronic fatigue syndrome	Non-specific muscular pain, all body affected

Page 19

In the following box list any other musculoskeletal or physical conditions (for example craniosacral imbalances) that can be associated with disorders in the systemic system. Indicate how the two, physical and visceral, are linked and how gross pathological causes of the symptoms are ruled out.

> Lower thoracic / upper lumbar problems affecting the gastrointestinal system through sympathetic outflow (thoracic chain) via cisterna chyli: no relation to food, no change to bowel habit
>
> Upper thoracic / low cervical problems affecting the stellate ganglion and blood flow to the cranium: neurological and other examinations normal

Page 20

Neoplasms can occur at any age and may be the cause of the patient's presenting complaint. If a neoplasm is present, what are the general signs / symptoms that may alert the practitioner?

> Generalised systemic symptoms of a neoplasm include unremitting pain, night pain, progressive pain and unexplained weight loss

Age	Named neoplasm	Typical presenting symptoms / signs
0-20	Ewing's tumour	Pain over tumour site, usually shaft of tibia
20-40	Testicular	Rapid enlargement of testis, or from site of secondary tumour
	Breast	Lump, nipple discharge, size change related to menstrual cycle
	Skin	
	Basal cell carcinoma	Slowly enlarging papule with central necrosis, usually on the face with a history of sun exposure
40-60	Lung	Cough, haemoptysis, dyspnoea, chest pain
	Breast	Lump, nipple discharge, size change related to menstrual cycle
	Bowel	Change in habits, flatus, bleeding, abdominal pain or mass
	Cervical	Abnormal vaginal bleeding or discharge, low back pain, dyspareunia, dysuria
	Skin	
	Squamous cell carcinoma	Keratotic nodules, exophylitic erythematous nodules, ulcers, with a firm edge
	Basal cell carcinoma	Slowly enlarging papule with central necrosis usually on the face with a history of sun exposure
	Malignant melanoma	Expanding, irregularly pigmented macule or plaque, with associated bleeding or crusting
60+	Prostate	Nocturia, hesitancy, poor stream, terminal dribbling
	Bowel	Change in habits, flatus, bleeding, abdominal pain or mass

2.4 Specific joint and joint complex signs and symptoms
2.4.1 Head and face
Page 22

Referral site / condition	How to determine from where the symptoms could be referred

Musculoskeletal referral
    Cervical spine
    Shoulder
	Symptoms aggravated / relieved by mobility of affected area / joint

Rheumatological condition
    Rheumatoid arthritis
    Systemic lupus erythematosus
    Sarcoidosis
	Associated systemic symptoms, specific pattern of symptoms, association with specific age, gender or race

Visceral referral
    Cardiovascular system
    (angina)
	Related to stress, age, exercise

Digestive system (hiatus hernia)	Related to food and posture after food

Page 23

What TMJ or other local musculoskeletal problem could give rise to head symptoms? In the following box list the conditions indicating the classical presenting symptom picture.

Degeneration of TMJ: limited jaw mobility (reduced opening), pain on chewing

What ear problems could give rise to head symptoms? In the following box list named conditions for the outer, middle and inner ear, indicating the classical presenting symptom picture.

Outer ear	Foreign body / blockage: parietal pain, deafness
Middle ear	Otitis media: child with fever, possible discharge
Inner ear	Menière's disease: dizziness, tinnitus

What facial and temporal problems could give rise to head symptoms? In the following box list any conditions (excluding the TMJ and cranial fascia) with their classical presenting symptom picture.

Temporal arteritis: related to polymyalgia rheumatica, pain / tenderness over temporal artery, no arterial pulse

What cranial vault or cranial fascia problems could give rise to head symptoms? In the following box list any conditions with their classical presenting symptom picture.

Brain tumour: headaches, mood swings, altered personality

Page 24

The four boxes below offer suggestions as to the cause of several common patterns of symptoms and do not attempt to cover the full range of causes for each symptom.

Age of onset of head or face symptoms

0-20	Trauma
20-40	Migraine
40-60	Glossopharyngeal, trigeminal neuralgia
60+	Hypertension

Site of head or face symptoms

Frontal	Sinus
Parietal	Constipation
Temporal	Migraine
Facial	Sinus
Occipital	Tension

Description of head or face symptoms

Throbbing pulsating	Vascular
Tight constricting band	Stress
Constant dull ache / pain	Trauma / injury

Pattern of head or face symptoms

Single episode	Trauma
Recurrent monthly	Migraine
Recurrent weekly	Migraine
Recurrent daily	Cluster
Night time	Intracranial disease, teeth grinding
Early morning	Hypertension
Afternoon / evening	Caffeine
Specific event(s)	Stress

2.4.1 Head and face

2.4.2 Cervical spine and cervicothoracic junction
Page 25

Referral site / condition	How to determine from where the symptoms could be referred

Musculoskeletal referral
    Shoulder complex
    Upper ribs / thorax
    Lumbar spine
	Symptoms aggravated / relieved by mobility of affected area / joint

Diaphragm	Related to breathing, rate, rhythm, underlying respiratory condition
Rheumatological condition Rheumatoid arthritis	Associated systemic symptoms, specific pattern of symptoms, association with specific age or gender

Visceral referral
    Cardiovascular system
    (shoulder, neck,
    upper thorax)
	Relation to stress, age, exercise

Biliary system (right shoulder)	Related to specific food, episodes of debilitating pain
Digestive system (retrosternal)	Related to food and posture after food

Page 26

0-20	Congenital	Kippel-Feil syndrome
	Developmental	Torticollis
	Rheumatological	Juvenile rheumatoid arthritis

20-40	Congenital	Cervical rib
	Developmental	Scoliosis
	Postural / occupational	Sedentary, repetitive movements
	Rheumatological	Rheumatoid arthritis

40-60	Hormonal / age	Osteoporosis, degeneration
	Postural / occupational	Sedentary, forward head posture, scoliosis
	Rheumatological	Ankylosing spondylitis

60+	Degenerative	Osteophytic formation, cervical bar
	Hormonal / age	Osteoporosis
	Rheumatological	Polymyalgia rheumatica

Page 27

Generally, musculoskeletal symptoms occur following a specific event or gradually for no apparent reason over a period of days, months or years.

If the onset was sudden, resulting from one notable incident, suggest causes for the patient's symptoms bearing in mind your experience.

1) Sudden movement of neck

2) Road traffic accident

For the above indicate the primary tissues causing symptoms, together with your personal differential diagnostic rationale for selecting those tissues (aggravating and relieving features).

1) Facet with overlying muscle spasm
Aggravating features: movement in specific directions; relieving features: other movement, rest, heat

2) Facet and ligamentous tissue with overlying muscle hypertonicity
Aggravating features: pain at limit of range; relieving features: heat, rest

Page 28

If the onset was for no apparent reason, suggest causes for the patient's symptoms bearing in mind your experience.

1) Posture at workstation / desk

2) Posture during leisure activity

For the above indicate the primary tissues causing symptoms, together with your personal differential diagnostic rationale for selecting those tissues (aggravating and relieving features).

1) Ligamentous tissue
Aggravating features: static posture, end of day; relieving features: mobility of neck, movement away from workstation / desk

2) Muscles (specific) or ligaments
Aggravating features: leisure activity (specific posture); relieving features: avoidance of specific posture

As the cervical spine is the final part of the spinal column, indicate what other musculoskeletal problems (either spinal or lower limb) could produce local cervical symptoms.

1) Pain in foot, causing a limp or altered posture, breakdown in final compensation in cervical spine

2) Short / long leg causing scoliosis to develop, degeneration in scoliosis leading to increasing lateral curves

2.4.3 Thoracic cage
Page 29

Referral site / condition	How to determine from where the symptoms could be referred
Musculoskeletal referral Shoulder	Symptoms aggravated / relieved by mobility of affected area / joint
Rheumatological condition Rheumatoid arthritis	Associated systemic symptoms, specific pattern of symptoms, association with specific age or gender

Visceral referral
    Cardiovascular system
    (left or right shoulder)
	Related to stress, age, exercise

Respiratory system (diaphragm [left or right shoulder])	Related to breathing, rate, rhythm, underlying respiratory condition
Biliary system (right shoulder)	Related to specific food, episodes of debilitating pain
Renal system (left or right loin)	Localised debilitating pain, haematuria

Other
    (left shoulder)
    (generalised)
	Splenomegaly, infection, haematological disorders
	History of psychiatric / psychogenic / anxiety problems, signs of cancer (unremitting pain, night pain, weight loss)

Page 30

Organ	Descriptive terms used to describe the pain
Heart	Crushing
Digestive (oesophagus)	Burning
Respiratory	Pain on breathing
Biliary	Colic

Site of pain	Referring organ or system
Retrosternal	Digestive (oesophagus) Cardiovascular
Chest wall	Neurological (Herpes zoster) Respiratory
Upper thoracic cage	Cardiovascular
Whole chest	Neurological (psychogenic) Any organ / system (advanced neoplasm)

Page 31

0-20	Congenital	Cervical rib
	Developmental	Scheuermann's disease
	Rheumatological	Reiter's syndrome

20-40	Congenital	Cervical rib
	Developmental	Scoliosis
	Postural / occupational	Sedentary, repetitive movements
	Rheumatological	Ankylosing spondylitis

40-60	Hormonal / age	Osteoporosis
	Postural / occupational	Scoliosis, increasing kyphosis
	Rheumatological	Polymyalgia rheumatica

60+	Degenerative	Spondylosis
	Hormonal / age	Osteoporosis
	Rheumatological	Polymyalgia rheumatica

Page 32

Generally, musculoskeletal symptoms occur following a specific event or gradually for no apparent reason over a period of days, months or years.

If the onset was sudden, resulting from one notable incident, suggest causes for the patient's symptoms bearing in mind your experience.

1) Trauma / fall

2) Sudden rotation

For the above indicate the primary tissues causing symptoms, together with your personal differential diagnostic rationale for selecting those tissues (aggravating and relieving features).

1) Facet (costovertebral or costochondral)
Aggravating features: movement, breathing, coughing; relieving features: support, splinting, compression

2) Spasm of the intercostal muscles / costovertebral joints
Aggravating features: contralateral side bending or ipsilateral rotation; relieving features: heat, rest

Page 33

If the onset was for no apparent reason, suggest causes for the patient's symptoms bearing in mind your experience.

1) Osteochondritic condition

2) Spondyloarthrosis causing increased kyphosis

For the above indicate the primary tissues causing symptoms, together with your personal differential diagnostic rationale for selecting those tissues (aggravating and relieving features).

1) Facets of adjoining areas, hypermobility
Aggravating features: movement; relieving features: rest, heat, support

2) Subchondral bone, hypertonia of muscles
Aggravating features: sustained posture; relieving features: gentle mobility

Indicate what spinal changes or named pathological conditions could occur in the thoracic spine of a postmenopausal woman or elderly male patient.

Osteoporosis

Polymyalgia rheumatica

Spinal fracture

2.4.4 Lumbar spine
Page 34

Referral site / condition	How to determine from where the symptoms could be referred

Musculoskeletal referral
    Pelvis
    Hip
	Symptoms aggravated / relieved by mobility of affected area / joint

Rheumatological condition Polymyalgia rheumatica	Prolonged morning stiffness, symptoms improve during day. Patient over 55 years, F>M

Visceral referral
    Cardiovascular system
    (abdominal aorta)
	Sudden onset symptoms, abdominal pulsations

Pelvic viscera	Menstrual abnormalities / amenorrhoea or vaginal discharge

Page 35

0-20	Congenital	Spina bifida
	Developmental	Spondylolisthesis
	Rheumatological	Ankylosing spondylitis

20-40	Congenital	Spina bifida
	Developmental	Spondylolisthesis
	Postural / occupational	Repetitive lifting
	Rheumatological	Ankylosing spondylitis

40-60	Hormonal / age	Osteoporosis
	Postural / occupational	Repetitive lifting, spondylolisthesis
	Rheumatological	Polymyalgia rheumatica

60+	Degenerative	Spondylosis, spondylolisthesis
	Hormonal / age	Osteoporosis
	Rheumatological	Polymyalgia rheumatica

Page 36

Generally, musculoskeletal symptoms occur following a specific event or gradually for no apparent reason over a period of days, months or years.

If the onset was sudden, resulting from one notable incident, suggest causes for the patient's symptoms bearing in mind your experience.

---

1) Bending and rotation, particularly in morning

2) Trauma / fall

For the above indicate the primary tissues causing symptoms, together with your personal differential diagnostic rationale for selecting those tissues (aggravating and relieving features).

---

1) Disc herniation or rupture of annulus fibrosus
Aggravating features: Valsalva manoeuvre, coughing / sneezing; relieving features: off weight-bearing, lying flat

2) Facet
Aggravating features: movement; relieving features: rest, support

---

Page 37

If the onset was for no apparent reason, suggest causes for the patient's symptoms bearing in mind your experience.

---

1) Spondylolisthesis

2) Spondyloarthrosis causing increased kyphosis

For the above indicate the primary tissues causing symptoms, together with your personal differential diagnostic rationale for selecting those tissues (aggravating and relieving features).

---

1) Ligament, annulus fibrosus, muscles
Aggravating features: prolonged, static, unsupported posture, long history from young age;
relieving features: mobility, support, rest, muscle strength

2) Subchondral bone, hypertonia of muscles
Aggravating features: sustained posture; relieving features: gentle mobility

---

Indicate what spinal changes or named pathological conditions could occur in the lumbar spine of a postmenopausal woman or elderly male patient.

Osteoporosis

Polymyalgia rheumatica

Secondary deposits from prostatic cancer

2.4.5 Pelvis
Page 39

Referral site / condition	How to determine from where the symptoms could be referred
Musculoskeletal referral Lumbar spine Hip	Symptoms aggravated / relieved by mobility of affected area / joint
Rheumatological condition Polymyalgia rheumatica	Prolonged morning stiffness, symptoms improve during day. Patient over 55 years, F>M
Ankylosing spondylitis	Bilateral pain, prolonged morning stiffness, reduced mobility
Visceral referral Pelvic viscera	Reproductive organs: menstrual abnormalities / amenorrhoea or vaginal discharge Prostate: nocturia, poor stream, terminal dribbling
Abdominal viscera	Changes in bowel habit, localised pain, swelling in groin

Page 40

0-20	Congenital	Lumbosacral bony abnormaility
	Developmental	Hypermobility due to activities
	Rheumatological	Ankylosing spondylitis

20-40	Congenital	Lumbosacral bony abnormaility
	Developmental	Cyclical problems (menstruation)
	Postural / occupational	Repetitive rotation movement
	Rheumatological	Ankylosing spondylitis

40-60	Hormonal / age	Fibrous fusion, osteoporosis
	Postural / occupational	Repetitive rotation movement
	Rheumatological	Polymyalgia rheumatica

60+	Degenerative	Osseous fusion
	Hormonal / age	Osteoporosis
	Rheumatological	Polymyalgia rheumatica

2.4.5 Pelvis

Page 41

Generally, musculoskeletal symptoms occur following a specific event or gradually for no apparent reason over a period of days, months or years.

If the onset was sudden, resulting from one notable incident, suggest causes for the patient's symptoms bearing in mind your experience.

Sacroiliac	Trip or fall, torsion through pelvis
Sacrococcygeal	Childbirth
Symphysis pubis	Sport

For the above indicate the primary tissues causing symptoms, together with your personal differential diagnostic rationale for selecting those tissues (aggravating and relieving features). Identify which joint(s) the condition will affect.

Sacroiliac	Ligaments - aggravating features: crossing legs, climbing stairs, twisting; relieving features: support, compression
Sacrococcygeal	Ligaments - aggravating features: sitting; relieving features: sitting on rubber ring
Symphysis pubis	Ligaments / muscles - aggravating features: contraction of adductors, rectus abdominus; relieving features: rest, support

Page 42

If the onset was for no apparent reason, suggest causes for the patient's symptoms bearing in mind your experience.

Sacroiliac	Short leg / long leg
Sacrococcygeal	Hyperflexion of coccyx
Symphysis pubis	Instability

For the above indicate the primary tissues causing symptoms, together with your personal differential diagnostic rationale for selecting those tissues (aggravating and relieving features). Identify which joint(s) the condition will affect.

Sacroiliac	Ligaments - aggravating features: crossing legs, prolonged standing; relieving features: support
Sacrococcygeal	Ligaments - aggravating features: sitting on a hard surface, hard chair; relieving features: sitting on a soft seat / cushion
Symphysis pubis	Ligaments - aggravating features: torsion through pelvis; relieving features: support, compression

2.4.6 Shoulder complex
Page 43

Referral site / condition	How to determine from where the symptoms could be referred
Musculoskeletal referral Cervical spine	Symptoms aggravated / relieved by mobility of affected area / joint
Rheumatological condition Rheumatoid arthritis	Associated systemic symptoms, specific pattern of symptoms, association with specific age or gender

Visceral referral
   Cardiovascular system
   (left or right shoulder)
	Related to stress, age, exercise

Respiratory system (diaphragm [left or right shoulder])	Related to breathing, rate, rhythm, underlying respiratory condition
Biliary system (right shoulder)	Related to specific food, episodes of debilitating pain
Other (left shoulder)	Splenomegaly, infection, haematological disorders

Page 44

0-20	Congenital	Shallow glenoid fossa
	Developmental	Dislocation
	Rheumatological	Rheumatoid arthritis

20-40	Congenital	Shallow glenoid fossa
	Developmental	Dislocation
	Postural / occupational	Recurrent dislocation
	Rheumatological	Rheumatoid arthritis

40-60	Hormonal / age	Supraspinatus degeneration / rupture
	Postural / occupational	Recurrent dislocation
	Rheumatological	Polymyalgia rheumatica

60+	Degenerative	Acromioclavicular degeneration
	Hormonal / age	Supraspinatus calcification / rupture
	Rheumatological	Polymyalgia rheumatica

Page 45

Generally, musculoskeletal symptoms occur following a specific event or gradually for no apparent reason over a period of days, months or years.

If the onset was sudden, resulting from one notable incident, suggest causes for the patient's symptoms bearing in mind your experience.

---

1) Impaction / compression of glenohumeral joint

2) Repetitive movement of glenohumeral joint

For the above indicate the primary tissues causing symptoms, together with your personal differential diagnostic rationale for selecting those tissues (aggravating and relieving features).

---

1) Bursa inflammation
Aggravating features: compression, painful arc of movement; relieving features: distraction, gentle mobility

2) Biceps tendonitis
Aggravating features: isotonic contraction of muscle; relieving features: rest, isometric contraction of muscle

---

Page 46

If the onset was for no apparent reason, suggest causes for the patient's symptoms bearing in mind your experience.

---

1) Adhesive capsulitis

2) Degeneration of acromioclavicular joint

For the above indicate the primary tissues causing symptoms, together with your personal differential diagnostic rationale for selecting those tissues (aggravating and relieving features).

---

1) Synovial membrane, muscles (rotator cuff)
Aggravating features: end of range of all movements, morning pain; relieving features: splinting of arm by body, rest

2) Subchondral bone
Aggravating features: movement of joint, compression of joint; relieving features: gentle traction, rest

---

2.4.7 Elbow joint complex
Page 47

Referral site / condition	How to determine from where the symptoms could be referred
Musculoskeletal referral	
Cervical spine	Symptoms aggravated / relieved by mobility of affected area / joint; neurological symptoms of a nerve root pattern
Thoracic outlet	Non-specific neurovascular and neurological symptoms
Rheumatological condition	
Rheumatoid arthritis	Associated systemic symptoms, specific pattern of symptoms, association with specific age or gender
Visceral referral	
Haemarthrosis	History of delayed or absence of blood clotting, warfarin medication

Page 48

0-20	Congenital	Cubitus valgus / varus
	Developmental	Dislocated radial head
	Rheumatological	Rheumatoid arthritis

20-40	Congenital	Cubitus valgus / varus
	Developmental	Loose bodies
	Postural / occupational	Pressure from leaning on surface
	Rheumatological	Rheumatoid arthritis, sarcoidosis

40-60	Hormonal / age	Loose bodies
	Postural / occupational	Tear of common flexor or extensor tendon
	Rheumatological	Rheumatoid arthritis

60+	Degenerative	Ulnar nerve entrapment
	Hormonal / age	Loose bodies
	Rheumatological	Rheumatoid arthritis

Page 49

Generally, musculoskeletal symptoms occur following a specific event or gradually for no apparent reason over a period of days, months or years.

If the onset was sudden, resulting from one notable incident, suggest causes for the patient's symptoms bearing in mind your experience.

> 1) Repetitive movements, tennis / golfer's elbow
>
> 2) Trauma in childhood

For the above indicate the primary tissues causing symptoms, together with your personal differential diagnostic rationale for selecting those tissues (aggravating and relieving features).

> 1) Musculotendinous junction or attachment onto bone
> Aggravating features: contraction of muscle, gripping thin handles; relieving features: rest, gripping thick handles
>
> 2) Annular ligament of radial head
> Aggravating features: use of arm especially supination / pronation; relieving features: rest, support

Page 50

If the onset was for no apparent reason, suggest causes for the patient's symptoms bearing in mind your experience.

> 1) Degeneration, osteophytic formation over ulnar groove
>
> 2) Enlarged fat pad / bursa

For the above indicate the primary tissues causing symptoms, together with your personal differential diagnostic rationale for selecting those tissues (aggravating and relieving features).

> 1) Neural tissue (ulnar nerve)
> Aggravating features: pressure on elbow; relieving features: extension of elbow, removal of pressure
>
> 2) Chronic inflammation of bursa or enlarged fat pad over the olecranon process
> Aggravating features: leaning on elbow, compression; relieving features: use, movement

There are three named nerves that can be compressed at various sites round the elbow. Name the nerve affected, the tissue causing the compression and area of the resultant neurological symptoms.

> Ulnar nerve - osteophytic encroachment of the ulnar groove (humerus) - lateral border of hand
>
> Radial nerve - supinator - dorsum of hand
>
> Median nerve - pronator teres - finger tips and thumb

2.4.8 Wrist and hand complex
Page 51

Referral site / condition	How to determine from where the symptoms could be referred

Musculoskeletal referral
   Elbow
   Cervical spine
	Symptoms aggravated / relieved by mobility of affected area / joint; neurological symptoms of a dermatonal / nerve root pattern

Rheumatological condition Rheumatoid arthritis	Associated systemic symptoms, specific pattern of symptoms, association with specific age or gender
Visceral referral Cardiovascular system	Related to stress, age, exercise
Respiratory system	Related to breathing, rate, rhythm, underlying respiratory condition
Endocrine system	Non-specific depending upon underlying condition

Page 52

0-20	Congenital	Madelung's deformity
	Developmental	Kienböcks osteochondritis
	Rheumatological	Rheumatoid arthritis

20-40	Congenital	Madelung's deformity
	Developmental	Volkmann's contracture
	Postural / occupational	Tenosynovitis
	Rheumatological	Rheumatoid arthritis, psoriatic arthropathy

40-60	Hormonal / age	Dupuytren's contracture, carpal tunnel syndrome
	Postural / occupational	Trigger finger
	Rheumatological	Rheumatoid arthritis, psoriatic arthropathy

60+	Degenerative	Osteoarthritis
	Hormonal / age	Dupuytren's contracture
	Rheumatological	Rheumatoid arthritis

Page 53

Generally, musculoskeletal symptoms occur following a specific event or gradually for no apparent reason over a period of days, months or years.

If the onset was sudden, resulting from one notable incident, suggest causes for the patient's symptoms bearing in mind your experience.

1) Forced extension or abduction of thumb

2) Fall / trauma

For the above indicate the primary tissues causing symptoms, together with your personal differential diagnostic rationale for selecting those tissues (aggravating and relieving features).

1) Articular cartilage, joint capsule, subchondral bone
Aggravating features: gripping, pressure through thumb; relieving features: support, gentle movement

2) Fracture of scaphoid or other carpal bone
Aggravating features: use, movement; relieving features: support, static position

Page 54

If the onset was for no apparent reason, suggest causes for the patient's symptoms bearing in mind your experience.

1) Carpal tunnel compression

2) Compression of ulnar nerve

For the above indicate the primary tissues causing symptoms, together with your personal differential diagnostic rationale for selecting those tissues (aggravating and relieving features).

1) Neural tissue (median nerve)
Aggravating features: morning pain or pins and needles, lateral aspect of hand;
relieving features: elevation of arm, movement of fingers

2) Neural tissue
Aggravating features: resting wrist when using computer mouse, riding bike / motor bike;
relieving features: removing pressure, mobility

Page 55

Rheumatological / connective tissue

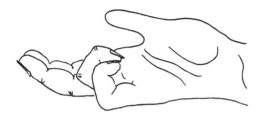

Dupuytren's contracture.

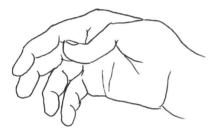

Rheumatotd arthritis deformity (affecting thumb).

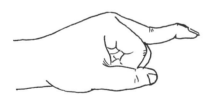

Swan neck deformity (seen in rheumatoid arthritis or after trauma).

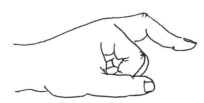

Boutonnière deformity (seen in rheumatoid arthritis or after trauma).

Neurological

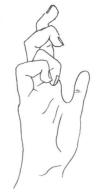

Bishop's hand (ulnar nerve palsy).

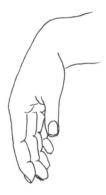

Wrist drop (radial nerve palsy).

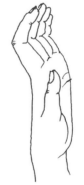

Ape hand (median nerve palsy).

Figure 2.1 Deformities in the hand and wrist.

2.4.9 Hip joint
Page 57

Referral site / condition	How to determine from where the symptoms could be referred
Musculoskeletal referral	
Psoas spasm	Symptoms aggravated by contraction / stretch of muscle
Pelvis	Symptoms aggravated / relieved by mobility of affected area / joint;
Lumbar spine	neurological symptoms of a dermatonal / nerve root pattern
Rheumatological condition	
Ankylosing spondylosis	Bilateral pain, prolonged morning stiffness, reduced mobility
Visceral referral	
Respiratory system	History of respiratory symptoms, cough, infection, underlying respiratory condition (tuberculosis)
Abdominal viscera	Presence of mass in groin or scrotum Inguinal hernia (direct or indirect)

Page 58

0-20	Congenital	Congenital dislocation of the hip
	Developmental	Perthes' disease, slipped femoral epiphysis
	Rheumatological	Rheumatoid arthritis (rare)

20-40	Congenital	Shallow acetabulum
	Developmental	Perthes' disease
	Postural / occupational	Early osteoarthritis
	Rheumatological	Sarcoidosis

40-60	Hormonal / age	Osteoporosis
	Postural / occupational	Osteoarthritis
	Rheumatological	Paget's disease, ankylosing spondylitis

60+	Degenerative	Osteoarthritis
	Hormonal / age	Osteoporosis, fracture of neck of femur
	Rheumatological	Polymyalgia rheumatica

Page 59

Generally, musculoskeletal symptoms occur following a specific event or gradually for no apparent reason over a period of days, months or years.

If the onset was sudden, resulting from one notable incident, suggest causes for the patient's symptoms bearing in mind your experience.

---

1) Trauma, fracture of femoral neck

2) Sudden contraction / stretch of muscle

For the above indicate the primary tissues causing symptoms, together with your personal differential diagnostic rationale for selecting those tissues (aggravating and relieving features).

---

1) Bone
Aggravating features: pressure, movement, weight-bearing; relieving features: rest, off weight-bearing

2) Muscle tissue
Aggravating features: contraction of specific muscle, specific movement; relieving features: heat, support, avoidance of specific movement

---

Page 60

If the onset was for no apparent reason, suggest causes for the patient's symptoms bearing in mind your experience.

---

1) Osteoarthritis

2) Trochanteric bursitis

For the above indicate the primary tissues causing symptoms, together with your personal differential diagnostic rationale for selecting those tissues (aggravating and relieving features).

---

1) Bone, subchondral bone
Aggravating features: pressure, weight-bearing; relieving features: sitting, rest, heat

2) Inflammation of bursa
Aggravating features: contraction of muscles over bursa, lying on side with compression of bursa; relieving features: decompression, lying on side with no pressure on bursa

---

2.4.10 Knee joint
Page 61

Referral site / condition	How to determine from where the symptoms could be referred

Musculoskeletal referral
    Hip joint
    Foot
	Symptoms aggravated / relieved by mobility of affected area / joint

Rheumatological condition Rheumatoid arthritis	Associated systemic symptoms, specific pattern of symptoms, association with specific age or gender
Visceral referral Haemarthrosis	History of delayed or absence of blood clotting, warfarin medication

Page 62

0-20	Congenital	Dislocation of patella
	Developmental	Chondromalacia patella
	Rheumatological	Rheumatoid arthritis

20-40	Congenital	Dislocation of patella
	Developmental	Osteochondritis dissecans
	Postural / occupational	Housemaid's knee, meniscoid tear
	Rheumatological	Reiter's syndrome

40-60	Hormonal / age	Osteoporosis
	Postural / occupational	Osteoarthritis, meniscoid tear
	Rheumatological	Rheumatoid arthritis, Paget's disease

60+	Degenerative	Osteoarthritis
	Hormonal / age	Osteoporosis
	Rheumatological	Rheumatoid arthritis

Page 63

Generally, musculoskeletal symptoms occur following a specific event or gradually for no apparent reason over a period of days, months or years.

If the onset was sudden, resulting from one notable incident, suggest causes for the patient's symptoms bearing in mind your experience.

1) Torn menisci (usually medial): extending the weight-bearing flexed knee with added rotation

2) Dislocation of patella

For the above indicate the primary tissues causing symptoms, together with your personal differential diagnostic rationale for selecting those tissues (aggravating and relieving features).

1) Subchondral bone, ligaments
Aggravating features: movement, weight-bearing; relieving features: rest, off weight-bearing, flexed knee

2) Subchondral bone, muscle spasm
Aggravating features: weight on flexed knee; relieving features: extension of knee (to allow patella to return to correct position)

Page 64

If the onset was for no apparent reason, suggest causes for the patient's symptoms bearing in mind your experience.

1) Loose body: osteochondritis dissecans

2) Overstrain of medial collateral ligament

For the above indicate the primary tissues causing symptoms, together with your personal differential diagnostic rationale for selecting those tissues (aggravating and relieving features).

1) Synovial membrane, subchondral bone
Aggravating features: movement, pressure; relieving features: rest, support

2) Ligamentous tissue
Aggravating features: weight-bearing, standing; relieving features: arch supports, gentle mobility

2.4.11 Ankle and foot complex
Page 65

Referral site / condition	How to determine from where the symptoms could be referred

Musculoskeletal referral
    Knee
    Lumbar spine
	Symptoms aggravated / relieved by mobility of affected area / joint; neurological symptoms of a dermatonal / nerve root pattern

Rheumatological condition Rheumatoid arthritis	Associated systemic symptoms, specific pattern of symptoms, association with specific age or gender
Reiter's syndrome	Young promiscuous male, conjunctivitis, urethritis
Visceral referral Abdominal viscera	Abdominal pain, altered stools (ulcerative colitis)

Page 66

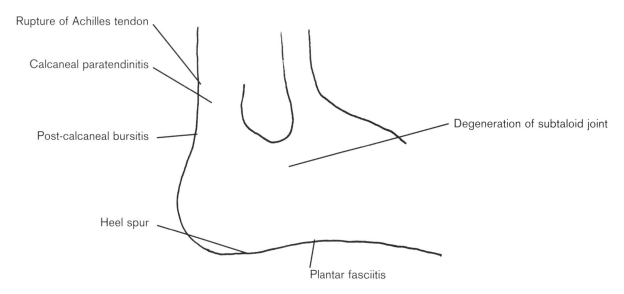

Rupture of Achilles tendon

Calcaneal paratendinitis

Post-calcaneal bursitis

Heel spur

Degeneration of subtaloid joint

Plantar fasciitis

Figure 2.2 Medial aspect of the ankle and rear foot.

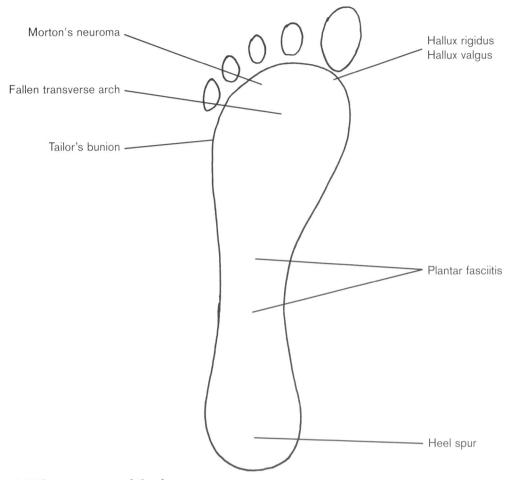

Morton's neuroma

Fallen transverse arch

Tailor's bunion

Hallux rigidus
Hallux valgus

Plantar fasciitis

Heel spur

Figure 2.3 Plantar aspect of the foot.

Page 67

0-20	Congenital	Talipes equinus / equinovarus
	Developmental	Köhler's disease (osteochondritis navicular)
	Rheumatological	Rheumatoid arthritis

20-40	Congenital	Pes cavus
	Developmental	Hindfoot varus / valgus
	Postural / occupational	Pes planus
	Rheumatological	Reiter's syndrome, ulcerative colitis

40-60	Hormonal / age	Gout
	Postural / occupational	Hallux valgus, dropped metatarsal heads
	Rheumatological	Ulcerative colitis

60+	Degenerative	Hallux rigidus
	Hormonal / age	Gout
	Rheumatological	Ulcerative colitis

Page 68

The foot is considered in relation to its three functional areas: the rearfoot and ankle, the midfoot and the forefoot.

Generally, musculoskeletal symptoms occur following a specific event or gradually for no apparent reason over a period of days, months or years.

If the onset was sudden, resulting from one notable incident, suggest causes for the patient's symptoms bearing in mind your experience.

Rearfoot and ankle	Midfoot	Forefoot
Inversion / eversion strain	Trauma, sport	Wearing high heels

For the above indicate the primary tissues causing symptoms, together with your personal differential diagnostic rationale for selecting those tissues (aggravating and relieving features).

Rearfoot and ankle	Midfoot	Forefoot
Ligaments Aggravating features: walking Relieving features: rest, compression, ice	Facet (cuboid) Aggravating features: walking, pressure Relieving features: rest	Subchondral bone Aggravating features: pressure on metartasal heads Relieving features: flat shoes, rest, supports

Page 69

If the onset was for no apparent reason, suggest causes for the patient's symptoms bearing in mind your experience.

Rearfoot and ankle	Midfoot	Forefoot
Calcaneal spur	Plantar fasciitis	Gout

For the above indicate the primary tissues causing symptoms, together with your personal differential diagnostic rationale for selecting those tissues (aggravating and relieving features).

Rearfoot and ankle	Midfoot	Forefoot
Subchondral bone, soft tissues of heel Aggravating features: pressure Relieving features: off weight-bearing, heel pad	Ligaments Aggravating features: prolonged stretch Relieving features: support of arch	Synovial membrane, joint structures Aggravating features: red wine, port, diet, pressure Relieving features: rest, care, no pressure

2.5 General health indicators and issues
Page 71

General health indicator	Underlying condition suggested
Weight	
Unexpected weight gain	Hypothyroid
Unexpected weight loss	Hyperthyroid, cancer
General health	
Fair	Generalised systemic disease
Poor	Generalised systemic disease
Always getting colds / flu	Poor immune system
Height	
Sudden loss of height	Crush fracture
Alcohol	
Female 14+ units per week	Liver disease
Male 21+ units per week	Liver disease
Smoking	Cardiovascular, respiratory, cancer
Recreational drugs	Tendency to psychiatric problems
Sensitivity to hot / cold	Thyroid

In the previous box various general health indicators are listed. List any other questions regarding their general health, or perception of general health that you would ask the patient. Indicate what aspects of their general health they are designed to investigate: physical and psychosocial.

Physical: bending, lifting

Psychosocial: care of child, strain on lifestyle, number of children / grandchildren

Page 72

Specific sign or predictor	Linked endocrine problem
Exceptionally large hands	Acromegaly
Size of neck	Hypothyroid (goitre)
Tremor	Hyperthyroid

Condition	Linked endocrine problem
Carpal tunnel syndrome	Hypothyroidism
Osteoporosis	Hyperparathyroidism, thyrotoxicosis, Cushing's disease
Muscle or bone pain	Cushing's disease, excessive anabolic steroids

Page 73

Two common endocrine problems that may become apparent when considering the patient's general health are related to insulin and thyroxine production. In the following three boxes list the common signs associated with abnormal production of these two hormones that may be identified when discussing the patient's general health.

Insulin and diabetes (type 2)

Obesity, hypertension, hyperlipidaemia, paraesthesia, pain, muscle weakness in legs, deterioration in vision, trophic brown scars on legs

Thyroxine and hypothyroidism

Fatigue, weight gain, cold intolerance, aches and muscle pains, anaemia, depression, constipation

Thyroxine and hyperthyroidism

Boundless energy, weight loss, heat intolerance, irritability, thirst, muscle weakness, diarrhoea

Page 74

System	Symptoms	Linked endocrine problem
Cardiovascular	Tachycardia Bradycardia	Type 1 or 2 diabetes, hyperthyroidism Hypothyroidism
Respiratory	Respiration rate	Type 1 diabetes, hypo / hyperthyroidism
Gastrointestinal	Diarrhoea / constipation	Hyperthyroidism, hypothyroidism, hyperparathyroidism
Neurological	Peripheral neuropathy Fine tremor	Type 1 and 2 diabetes, hyperthyroidism, hypoparathyroidism
Urinary	Polyuria	Type 1 diabetes, hyperparathyroidism
Reproductive	Infertility	Hypo / hyperthyroidism

2.6 Past medical history indicators and issues
2.6.1 Cardiovascular system
Page 76
Note in the box below three different questions that may uncover an underlying cardiovascular condition.

---

1) Do you ever feel a rapid, unexplained heart beat?

2) Are you ever breathless at night?

3) Do you get a pain in the chest on exertion?

Common cardiovascular conditions	Associated symptoms
Stable angina	Pain on effort
Deep vein thrombosis	Pain / tender calf Rapid swelling in leg Pitting, oedema, mild fever
Intermittent claudication	Walk for set distance before rest, then walk same distance

Page 77
In a very general way use the following box to indicate how these identified common cardiovascular conditions might affect a patient's posture, activities or lifestyle. Speculate how these changes may generate musculoskeletal symptoms and suggest a very general treatment plan (aims and objectives) that would assist this patient.

Reduced activity, reduced exercise

Generates musculoskeletal problems: poor muscle tone, poor support of musculoskeletal system, posture

Treatment plan: gentle mobility, exercise routines to improve muscle strength, tone and improve mobility, thus improving cardiovascular activity

---

2.6.2 Respiratory system
Page 78
Note in the box below three different questions that may uncover an underlying respiratory condition.

---

1) Do you get breathless when walking?

2) Do you have bouts of prolonged coughing?

3) Have you ever coughed up blood?

Common respiratory conditions	Associated symptoms
Asthma	Intermittent dyspnoea, coughing, wheezing
Chronic obstructive pulmonary disease	Chronic productive cough, dyspnoea, wheezing
Bronchiectasis	Persistent cough, copious purulent sputum

Page 79
In a very general way use the following box to indicate how these identified common respiratory conditions might affect a patient's posture, activities or lifestyle. Speculate how these changes may generate musculoskeletal symptoms and suggest a very general treatment plan (aims and objectives) that would assist this patient.

Reduced mobility of the ribs and thoracic cage

Generates musculoskeletal problems: hypertonia of secondary muscles of respiration

Treatment plan: improve mobility of thoracic cage, reduce tone of the muscles

---

2.6.3 Gastrointestinal system
Page 80
Note in the box below three different questions that may uncover an underlying gastrointestinal condition.

---

1) Have you noticed any change in bowel habit?

2) Have you noticed any bleeding from the rectum?

3) Do you get any pain when eating?

Common gastrointestinal conditions	Associated symptoms
Hiatus hernia	Retrosternal pain related to food and straining / stooping over after food
Cholestasis	Pain increased by eating fatty food, acute colic pain
Crohn's disease	Diarrhoea, abdominal pain, weight loss

Page 81
In a very general way use the following box to indicate how these identified common digestive conditions might affect a patient's posture, activities or lifestyle. Speculate how these changes may generate musculoskeletal symptoms and suggest a very general treatment plan (aims and objectives) that would assist this patient.

Reduced activity as eating frequently to reduce pain, increased weight due to over-eating.

Generates musculoskeletal problems: associated with weight increase, pressure on joints, increases degeneration

Treatment plan: improve mobility of hips and knees to encourage bending with back straight, increase exercise, advice regarding eating and diet

2.6.4 Neurological system
Page 83

Note in the box below three different questions that may uncover an underlying neurological condition is present.

---

1) Do you ever feel any tingling or weakness in the arms or legs?

2) Do you have any loss of sensation anywhere in the body?

3) Do you suffer from headaches?

Common neurological conditions	Associated symptoms
Herpes zoster	Severe unilateral, intercostal / face pain followed by vesicular rash
Transient ischaemic attack	Variable depending on the area affected. Can include muscle weakness / numbness, dysphagia, dysarthria
Migraine	Aura, unilateral throbbing headache, vomiting, photophobia

Page 84

In a very general way use the following box to indicate how these identified common neurological conditions might affect a patient's posture, activities or lifestyle. Speculate how these changes may generate musculoskeletal symptoms and suggest a very general treatment plan (aims and objectives) that would assist this patient.

Altered use of limbs, due to neglect or loss of sensation

Generates musculoskeletal problems: asymmetrical use of other unaffected limbs increases strain on other joints

Treatment plan: improve mobility of affected limbs to improve proprioception and to encourage symmetrical use of limbs

---

2.6.5 *Urinary and reproductive systems*
Page 85

Urinary system

Have you ever noticed any change in flow of urine?

Reproductive / gynaecological system

Have you ever had any gynaecological problems?

Note in the box below two simple questions that could be asked to identify the presence of an underlying urinary (not prostate) or reproductive disorder.

---

1) Have you experienced any pain or stinging on passing urine?

2) Have you experienced any spotting mid-cycle?

In the next box write down a general question that would, without embarrassment to the patient, give you an indication of the degree of any prostatic hypertrophy present.

Have you noticed a difficulty in starting or stopping the passage of urine?

Page 86

Common urinary conditions	Associated symptoms
Non-gonococcal urethritis	Thin discharge, cervicitis, urethritis, salpingitis
Prostatic hyperplasia	Over 60 years old, reduced urine flow, difficulty starting / stopping, urine retention in bladder

Common gynaecological conditions	Associated symptoms
Fibroids	Heavy painful menses
Endometriosis	Cyclical pain, bleeding, diarrhoea / constipation, low back ache

Page 87

In a very general way use the following box to indicate how these identified common conditions might affect a patient's posture, activities or lifestyle. Speculate how these changes may generate musculoskeletal symptoms and suggest a very general treatment plan (aims and objectives) that would assist this patient.

Urinary
Inability to venture out due to perceived need to be near toilet

Generates musculoskeletal problems: poor tone due to lack of exercise, feeling of isolation

Treatment plan: encourage development of pelvic floor muscles, boost self-confidence, improve mobility generally

Gynaecological
Tension via the three paired cervical ligaments (pubocervical, transverse cervical and sacrocervical)

Generates musculoskeletal problems: low back pain

Treatment plan: improve mobility in pelvis, sacroiliac and symphysis pubis, to reduce effect of tension through ligaments, improve pelvic floor tone to add extra support

2.6.6 *Ear, nose and throat*
Page 88

Note in the box below one simple question for each area that might uncover an underlying ear, nose and throat condition.

Ear	Have you experienced any dizziness or ringing in the ears?
Nose	Have you experienced any pain under the eyes?
Throat	Have you experienced frequent sore throats?

Common ear problems	Associated symptoms
Menière's disease	Recurrent spontaneous attacks of vertigo, hearing loss, tinnitus
Acute otitis media	Child or infant, signs of infection, possible perforation

Page 89

Common nose problems	Associated symptoms
Sinus infection	Pain over the affected sinus, spontaneous mucopurulent nasal discharge
Epistaxis	Linked with hypertension, trauma, acute nasal inflammatory process

Common throat problems	Associated symptoms
Exudative tonsillitis	Pain on swallowing may be an early symptom of glandular fever in teenagers or young adults
Dysphagia	Symptoms from pathology of respiratory tract, history of smoking

Page 90

In a very general way use the following box to indicate how these identified common ear, nose or throat conditions might affect a patient's posture, activities or lifestyle. Speculate how these changes may generate musculoskeletal symptoms and suggest a very general treatment plan (aims and objectives) that would assist this patient.

Holds head to one side or rotated to present good ear towards origin of sound
Generates musculoskeletal problems: added strain on cervical spine and muscles
Treatment plan: improve mobility of cervical and thoracic spine, encourage use of hearing aid

3.1 Observation

Section 3 Evaluation
3.1 Observation
Page 93

Once the patient is stripped to their underwear and you begin the normal physical evaluation, many signs, often of systemic disease, can be observed, from varicose veins to surgical scars. On Figure 3.1 indicate where you would expect to see scars for the named operations.

Appendix   Caesarean   Carpal tunnel   Gall bladder
Heart   Hip replacement   Hysterectomy   Knee cartilage
Kidney   Laparoscopy   Lumbar disc   Varicose veins

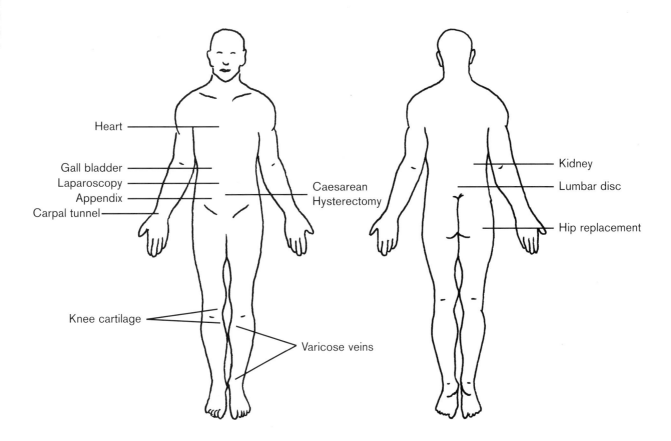

Figure 3.1 Outline of the body: anterior and posterior.

Page 94

Signs	Suggesting
Male wearing incontinence pants	Prostate problem
Obvious urine stains on underwear	Incontinence or prostate problem
Female wearing panty liners	Weak pelvic floor Post-menopausal bleeding
Blood on underwear	Haemorrhoids Post-menopausal bleeding

Multiple scars on forearms	Avid gardener Self-harm Careless cook (burns to wrist) Kittens at home
A dirty brown discoloration to the ankles and feet	Poor circulation
A yellowish tinge to the skin	Jaundice

Page 95

The patient suffers with psoriasis. How is this observed skin complaint related to joint pain?

Psoriatic arthopathy affects 10% of patients with psoriasis

Are there any other dermatological signs that may suggest an underlying systemic or musculoskeletal condition?

Reduced hair growth on legs / feet: cardiovascular

Erythema nodosum: rheumatological

Tuft of hair (lumbar spine): spina bifida occulta

Whilst generally observing the patient, a note of the depth, rate and rhythm of respiration can be made. What observations would suggest that a respiratory or cardiovascular examination is necessary?

Reduced depth	Bronchial spasm / obstruction
Increased rate	Reduced functional lung capacity
Rhythm	Poor oxygenation of blood, blood pooling in lungs

Page 96

Site	Signs	System(s) incriminated
Skin		
General	Thin / papery	Cardiovascular
Abdomen / thorax)	Dilated veins (round umbilicus)	Cardiovascular, biliary
Hands / fingers	Clubbing Peripheral cyanosis Janeway lesions	Respiratory, cardiovascular, digestive Cardiovascular, respiratory Cardiovascular
Feet / ankles	Peripheral cyanosis	Cardiovascular

Aspect	Feature	Endocrine condition
Skin	Scar (colour)	Cushing's disease
	Excessive / minimal perspiration	Thyroid
Hair (changes from normal)	Greasy / very dry	Thyroid
Nails (changes from normal)	Fragile	Thyroid

3.2 Palpation
Page 97

General sign	System	Reason
Temperature		
Very localised change	Musculoskeletal	Localised inflammatory response
Regional change	Cardiovascular	Raynaud's phenomenon
General increase / decrease	Cardiovascular	Poor blood supply legs, varicose veins
Oedema		
Pitting	Cardiovascular	Fluid collects in interstitial space
Non-pitting	Endocrine	Infiltration of mucopolysaccharide
	Musculoskeletal	Localised inflammatory response

Section 4 Specific system examination
4.1 Cardiovascular system examination

Page 99

During your observation and palpation of the patient you are alert to specific signs of cardiovascular disease. In the following box briefly list these signs.

> The colour and temperature of the skin, rate of breathing

4.1.1 Auscultation

When conducting auscultation of the heart it is noticed that the apex beat is not in the 5th intercostal space in the mid-clavicular line. What medical conditions could cause this change in position?

> Enlarged heart due to cardiovascular disease
> Enlarged heart due to over-exercise

Page 100

What structural conditions may cause the same finding?

> Marked structural scoliosis

4.1.2 Percussion

In the following box indicate what information you gain from percussing the heart.

> Size of heart, position of heart (very little else)

Why is the abdomen palpated?	Abdominal aorta
What palpatory findings would indicate an abnormality of this vital artery?	Lateral pulsations
Why is the abdomen percussed?	Ascites
What findings would indicate an abnormality?	Dull on percussion, area affected changes when the patient moves

4.1.3 Measurement of blood pressure
Page 101

This is a very common and simple procedure to undertake that, it could be argued, should be conducted on every patient. What are the arguments, both for and against, this point of view?

> For: good practice as it identifies pre-clinical hypertension, enables monitoring of condition and highlights a possible problem
>
> Against: this is not a therapist's area of responsibility, as they are treating holistically; may unduly alarm patient

How can you make an assessment of a patient's systolic blood pressure if your stethoscope is missing?

> Pump up the sphygmomanometer and palpate the radial pulse. This gives an indication of systolic pressure

How can you make an assessment of a patient's blood pressure if your sphygmomanometer is broken?

> Look in their eyes for nipping of veins by arteries. This gives an indication of high blood pressure

4.2 Respiratory system examination
Page 102

During your observation and palpation of the patient, you are alert to specific signs of respiratory disease. In the following box briefly list these signs.

Breathing pattern / rate / rhythm, colour of lips, cough

4.2.1 Auscultation

Adventitious breath sounds (description)	Never over normal lungs, can originate from pleura or pericardium Sounds added to normal breath sounds
Discontinuous breath sounds (description)	Pulmonary oedema, pneumonia, pulmonary fibrosis, Crackles - fine or coarse
Continuous breath sounds (description)	Asthma, obstructive disease Wheezes
Lack of breath sounds (description)	Consolidation / tumour No sound

Page 103

Voice sounds enhanced because	Consolidation of lungs
Voice sounds absent because	Voice too quiet (whispering)

4.2.2 Percussion

Sound	Underlying condition
Flatness	Pleural effusion
Dullness	Lobar pneumonia
Resonance	Bronchitis
Hyper-resonance	Emphysema
Tympany	Large pneumothorax

4.3 Gastrointestinal system examination

Page 104

During your observation and palpation of the patient you are alert to specific signs of gastrointestinal disease. In the following box briefly list these signs.

> Pulsations in the abdomen, dilated abdominal veins

4.3.1 Auscultation

Noise heard	Causes
No sound	Obstruction
Fluid 'sploshing' around	Ascites
Hyper-resonance	Air
Peritoneal rub	Peritonitis

4.3.2 Percussion

> What important structures can you identify when percussing the abdomen?
> Liver and stomach
>
> In addition to air, what features / conditions can you identify when percussing the abdomen?
> Ascites

4.3.3 Palpation

Page 105

Palpation is a vital tool when trying to identify abdominal structures. In the following box explain why palpation should begin away from any identified tender areas.

> For patient comfort and relaxation of the abdominal wall, as you move towards the tender area

Light palpation	Liver, large bowel, bladder (full)
Deep palpation	Diaphragm, aorta, pancreas

> Name the vital pulsating structure that should always be palpated in the abdomen.
> Aorta
>
> Where is the pulsation palpated in relation to the umbilicus?
> Superior to umbilicus
>
> In which direction is the pulsation normally detected (anteriorly or laterally)?
> Anterior
>
> What clinical emergency may be suggested if the pulsation is increased or displaced laterally?
> Aortic aneurysm

4.4 Neurological system examination
Page 107

During your observation of the patient you are alert to specific signs of neurological disease. In the following box briefly list these signs.

> Fasciculation of muscle, wasting of muscle, cuts / burns on skin (no memory of injury)

4.4.1 Palpation

Neurological conditions	Muscle tone	Sensory signs
Multiple sclerosis	Spastic weakness	Variable loss
Peripheral neuropathy	Distal weakness	Glove / stocking loss
Bell's palsy	Unilateral weakness of face	Normal
Cerebrovascular accident	Spasticity of affected side	Impaired positional sense. Reduction of pain and sense of light touch on affected side
Peripheral nerve lesion	Specific muscle weakness	Specific sensory loss, paraesthesia
Parkinson's disease	Resting tremor Cog-wheel rigidity	Normal

4.4.2 Sensory neurological examination
Page 108

A sensory neurological loss will have an obvious effect upon how the patient perceives external stimuli. In the following box describe your routine for identifying the extent of sensory loss and how you would test for it.

> Begin in the area of sensory loss, work out in all directions to normal sensation area. The areas of sensory loss can be mapped by pinprick, light touch or by vibration

Loss	Indicating
Vibration sense	Peripheral neuropathy
Light touch	Peripheral nerve
Pinprick	Peripheral nerve

Page 109

Condition	Area of sensory / joint positional loss	How tested
Nerve root lesion	Nerve root distribution	Sensory, reflexes
Peripheral nerve lesion	Cutaneous nerve distribution	Sensory, reflexes
Diabetic neuropathy	Glove / stocking distribution	Vibration 128Mhz, sensory, reflexes
Dorsal column lesion	Joint position sensation loss	Passive position of joint
Cerebrovascular accident	Variable depending on the area affected	Reflexes, passive movement of joint

Page 110
Figure 4.1 indicates the anterior and posterior dermal distribution of the spinal nerve roots to the upper and lower extremity. Identify and label the nerve root that supplies the areas demarcated by the dotted lines.

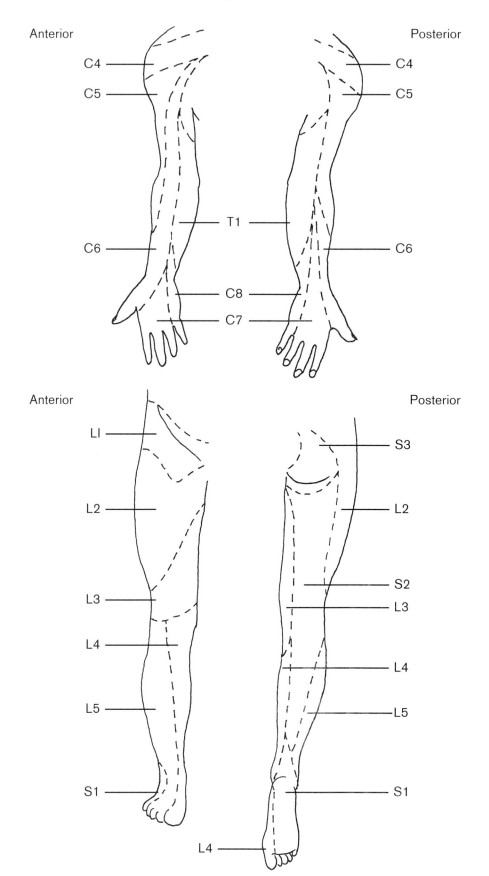

Figure 4.1 Anterior and posterior dermal distribution of the spinal nerve root.

Page 111

Figure 4.2 indicates the anterior and posterior dermal distribution of the peripheral nerves to the upper and lower extremity. Identify the peripheral nerves that supply the areas demarcated by the dotted lines.

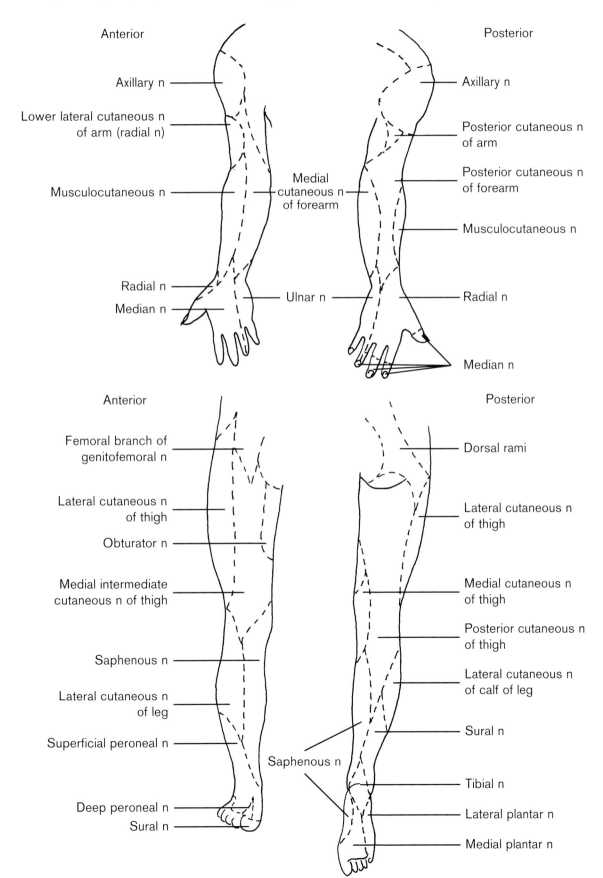

Figure 4.2 Anterior and posterior dermal distribution of the peripheral nerves.

4.4.3 Motor neurological examination
Page 112

The testing of reflexes are regularly carried out in the consulting room. Briefly describe how the deep muscular reflex works.

Stretch of muscle, stimulation muscle spindle, nerve signal to spinal cord, signal to contract muscle, muscle contraction. Response reduced by upper centres

Maxillary - Cranial nerve V	Patella - L2 / 3 / 4
Biceps - C5 / 6	Achilles - S1 / 2
Triceps - C6 / 7 / 8	
Brachioradialis (periosteoradial) - C5 / 6	

Several reflexes disappear in childhood. Name and briefly describe these infantile reflexes.

Sucking and swallowing, grasping, rooting, tonic neck

Plantar reflex	Stroke the sole of the foot causing the toes to dorsiflex
Gordon's finger sign	Apply pressure over the pisiform causing extension of flexed fingers
Hoffmann's sign	Flick the relaxed distal phalanx causing clawing of hand
McCarthy's sign	Percussion of the supra-orbital ridge causing constant blinking

Page 113

If the neurological damage was in a specific peripheral nerve, what muscle power findings would be present?

> Power of muscles supplied diminished, specific pattern

If the neurological damage was in a specific spinal nerve root, what muscle power findings would be present?

> Power of muscles supplied diminished, specific pattern

If the neurological damage was in the spinal cord or above, what muscle power findings would be present?

> There would be no muscle power below the level of the lesion, generalised pattern

Page 114

Spinal level	Resisted movement	Spinal level	Resisted movement
C1	Flexion of the neck	L2	Flexion of the hips
C2	Extension of the neck	L3	Extension of the knee
C3	Sidebend of the neck	L4	Dorsiflexion of the ankle
C4	Shrug of the shoulders	L5	Extension of the hallux
C5	Shoulder abduction	S1	Plantar flexion of the ankle
C6	Flexion of the elbow		
C7	Extension of the elbow		
C8	Flexion of the fingers		
T1	Abduction / adduction of the fingers		

Cranial nerve	Test	Abnormal findings
I	Smell	No smell
II	Visual / sight	Reduced visual field
III	Eye movement	Ptosis
IV	Eye movement	Diplopia
V	Open mouth	Jaw deviates to side
VI	Eye movement	Diplopia
VII	Whistle / raise eyebrow	Unable to whistle, weakness / droop
VIII	Hearing	Deafness / reduced hearing
IX	Gag	Palate pulled to side (rare)
X	Gag	Palate pulled to side
XI	Trapezius contraction	Weakness
XII	Tongue protrusion	Deviates to side

Page 115

Upper sign		Lower sign
Increased	Peripheral reflexes	Reduced
Normal	Specific muscle weakness (single nerve supply)	Present
Present	Limb tremor	Absent
Absent	Muscle fasciculation	Present
Present	Impaired coordination / balance	Absent
Present	General muscle weakness (multiple nerve supply)	Absent
Present (gross)	Altered gait	Present (local)
Absent	Joint position sense	Present
Increased	Involuntary resistance to joint movement	Absent
Present	Pathological reflex present	Absent
Absent	Infantile reflex present in infant	Present
Present	Glove stocking paraesthesia / numbness	Absent
Present	Infantile reflex present in child / adult	Absent
Absent	Dermatomal paraesthesia / numbness	Present
Absent	Stereognosis / graphaesthesia	Present
Absent	Vibration sense	Present